GO AN
EXTRA MILE

Michael Wood was born in 1919, and educated at Winchester and the Middlesex Hospital. He became a general surgeon and – having emigrated to East Africa after the Second World War – later a plastic surgeon.

In 1958, together with Sir Archibald McIndoe and Dr Thomas Rees of America, he founded the African Medical and Research Foundation, of which he is now Director General. In 1977 he was awarded the CBE for his work.

To Susan

GO AN EXTRA MILE

*The adventures and reflections
of a flying doctor*

MICHAEL WOOD
Foreword by Laurens van der Post

'And whosoever shall compel thee to go a
mile, go with him twain.'

St Matthew, Ch. 5, V. 41

Collins
FOUNT PAPERBACKS

First published in Great Britain by
William Collins Sons & Co Ltd, London, 1978

First issued in Fount Paperbacks, 1980

© Michael Wood 1978

Made and printed in Great Britain by
William Collins Sons & Co Ltd, Glasgow

Contents

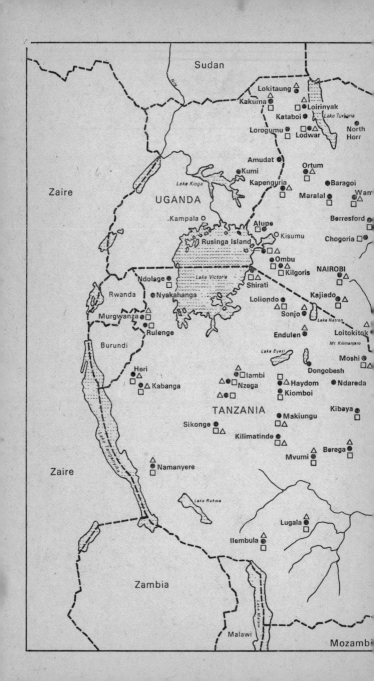

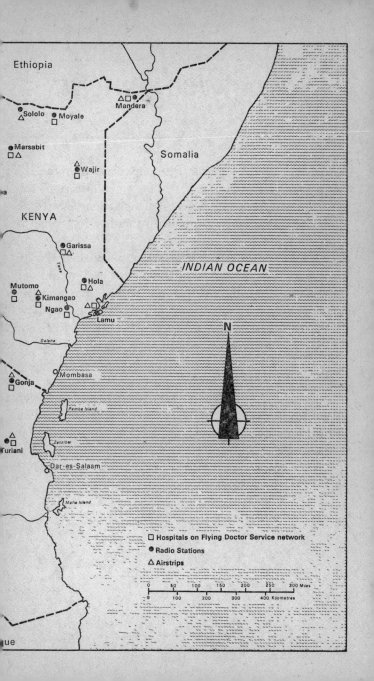

Acknowledgements

This is a book of personal reminiscences over the last thirty years in Africa and is in no way a history of the African Medical and Research Foundation (AMREF). This task awaits a more objective author sometime in the future.

It is not possible to thank all those people individually who have helped me over the years but I would, in particular, like to mention my wife, Susan, and my family, who have acted as my memory and been so long suffering; my colleagues everywhere in the African Medical and Research Foundation without whom there would have been little to tell; my friends at Ol Molog and in the bush in Africa.

I owe a special debt to my friend Laurens van der Post for writing the foreword and my secretary Pauline Ravn for typing the manuscript.

Foreword

Kipling, who made the most of anything that came his way, once wrote something which stayed unbidden with me while reading the manuscript of *Go An Extra Mile*. In a letter to the author of *The Cruise of the Cachalot*, a great deep-sea book which he had found 'immense', Kipling observed, not without unconscious envy, of a largesse of first-hand experience of which he himself was incapable: 'You have thrown away enough material to make five books and I congratulate you most heartily.' I cite Kipling in Michael's Wood's regard neither to compare nor to complain but as evidence of how greedy his book made me and how I finished my first reading of his manuscript longing and hoping for more.

Go An Extra Mile of course is autobiographical and, at a moment when taste in reading tends to reject fantasy and fiction and even objective history for living and immediate experience, that fact alone induces an instant appeal. Indeed, the book contains enough of the quintessentials of a life which is still being lived in its own unique end, in circumstances unusual even for Africa, to place it apart from the distinctive run of a crowded autobiographical field, and to make it for me one of the most important books to have come out of my native continent for many years.

This significance is of an unusually complex, many-sided and rounded kind and defies adequate analysis, let alone definition, in a mere foreword. But the key to a proper appreciation of its quality is to be found, I believe, in the impressive witness it bears to the knack Africa has of creating a special bond or contract without clause of escape, not only between it and those born to it but also with the many who come to it from without – careers predetermined and characters already set.

This remarkable phenomenon has had so marked a bearing on the history of Africa and is of such importance to its future, that it concerns me still today as it did at the beginning of my working life. Almost from the moment of leaving school, I was compelled on a world beat wider and larger than most. Yet not even so intensive a course in travel has revealed, with the qualified exception perhaps of India, any other land which could bend to its own dark and enigmatic earth the lives of such diversities and numbers of strangers from without, particularly those out of the Western World and most especially the 'Red Strangers' from Britain.

The proportions of this affair between Africa and the external world, in fact, assumed in time those of a mystery inviting trespass on preserves forbidden to a lawful pen. All one can say with justice and clarity is that there is much more to it than the compost heap of discarded motives like a lust after spice and gold, greed of traders and industrialists, fanaticism of missionaries and overlordly ambitions of world powers, that the slanted, clichéd and fashionably simplistic view of history would make of it. Besides, the makings of the affair have their origin in a time when none of these elements applied.

There are already indications of its existence far back in the animated gossip of Herodotus, in the strange compulsion which made a Greek traveller break his journey home from India and go up and out into the blue of East Africa to bring back to the pre-Christian Mediterranean news of snow – miraculous under the perpendicular sun of the equator, and of mountains so high and remote that Ptolemy designated them as of the moon. There is the evidence of the Roman Scipio Africanus's well-worn aside: 'Out of Africa something always new.' And nearer our own day there is the profoundly four-dimensional remark of the great Elizabethan physician of Norwich, Thomas Browne: 'We carry within us the worlds we seek without us,' he wrote, coming nearer the source of what is of mystery in the matter than anyone before or since. 'There is all Africa and her prodigies in us.'

From that Elizabethan moment, synchronized to the re-awakening of Europe with a finesse which cannot just be dismissed as idle, the testimony multiplies in the lives of all sorts and conditions of men, and this peculiar power of Africa gathers dominion over the imagination of Europe.

There never has been a continent to match Africa for lifting the most ordinary of lives out of the ordinary and, in Milton's great poetic phrase, to 'make men scorn delight and live laborious days'.

As a result I found myself reading this book as if in the company of all the 'extraordinary' ordinary people who made the vanishing Africa I knew as a boy, rather than that of the only too ordinary men in the high places and positions that enabled them to hog the perfunctory histories and official reports which crowd the shelves of our libraries and archives.

But ultimately the impact of the book is all the more meaningful because it is an answer to all legitimate doubt about the reality and future of this bond. Even I, who am of a family so utterly of the earth of Africa, have had agonizing doubts as to whether this bond between Africa and Europe in its deepest sense could survive the immense changes – the cruel and often sordid twists of fate inflicted on Africa since the last World War, and

I am certain that history will increasingly turn its attention towards a reappraisal of these aspects of the post-War years and examine the extent to which the transformation of Empire and Commonwealth was accomplished in a manner that defeated its own highest motivations, making of it not an act of emancipation so much as a self-inflicted wound, and a betrayal of what had become a trust of history and wards held in its chancery before coming of age.

But in regard to Africa, particularly this most beautiful and evocative part of it in which Michael Wood lives, his story left me strangely reassured. I found that *Go An Extra Mile* was not a title so much as an exhortation to the spirit apprenticed to Africa to achieve whatever might be needed to make this ancient land immediate and contemporary.

High as this claim may appear to be pitched, the story does indicate it convincingly because it circumscribes the full historic round of all the phases of this special relationship between Africa and the imagination of the Western World, particularly of Britain : the past, the tumultuous present and intimation of the future free of yesterday's negations.

The story begins inevitably with Michael Wood's beautiful wife Susan, an inspired maker of new homes, a writer, poet, artist, farmer and woman of action without loss of femininity. She was born deep in the old Congo of a father turned missionary, against all his education and family preconceptions, and a mother of Pre-Raphaelite beauty and temperament. She spent barely a year in the Congo but that year contained a horrific journey which took them from beyond the source of the White Nile, first with porters and then by sluggish river steamer, to its outlet on the Mediterranean. Such a journey, despite infections and malnutrition, failed to kill her spirit and proved enough to bind her to Africa for good. This was the decisive influence which made Michael Wood, newly qualified in medicine, and Sue, decide to emigrate from England to Kenya immediately after the War.

Kenya was still a British colony, confident, mature at last after participation in a second World War, and with an élan and style not to be found elsewhere in Commonwealth or Empire. But soon the brutal onslaught of the unbridled forces of change stormed down on them, and compelled them into areas of mind, being and behaviour without any outside examples or experience to instruct them, as in that strange, tragic, still uncomprehended and last of all Britain's colonial wars, known as Mau Mau and the era of Uhuru which followed so quickly with an instant success that was undeniable, however enigmatic its implications for the future.

I was associated with them in significant aspects of their lives throughout all these traumatic years and am witness of how they transcended one unprecedented crisis and turmoil after the other. They did so well, I believe, because both of them all their lives had foreseen change and recognized the urgent necessity of a renewal of men and their societies everywhere on earth.

For instance, they joined a small group of us of all races, creeds and colours, to try and prepare what was left of British Africa for a post-Colonial evolution towards a greater community of life which would freely abandon the race, class, religious and ideological discriminations which had so dangerously fragmented it in the past and so prevent, from lack of a transcendent social vision, the disintegration which would otherwise follow, as it has done in so many places.

I could not improve on Michael Wood's vivid, dramatic, frank, handwoven presentation of the main events of his life as, for instance, private surgeon, self-taught pilot, navigator for his son-in-law in one hair-raising East African Safari Rally after the other, and above all as co-founder of the African Medical and Research Foundation, which is popularly and proudly known everywhere as the Flying Doctor Service. I can cite perhaps only one phase of their lives to do service for all these others, because it seems to me to be a kind of parable of their lives.

Defeated in her efforts to work for East Africa also politically, and with Michael engaged in a desperate battle to keep the Flying Doctor Service alive, quite apart from transforming it into the great, unique, complex and widespread instrument of healing, not only in East Africa but across its frontiers with other states, which today it has become, Sue renewed the pattern of her own life as well. She decided that it was necessary for a proper balance in the lives of themselves and their children to go farming. They accordingly left Kenya, became citizens of Tanzania and, while Michael took medicine to the widely scattered and uncared for millions rather than try to bring them to the few and remote centralized hospitals, Sue established a new home on the steep flanks of Kilimanjaro. The Maasai name for the exact place sounded like a Tolkien incantation. Ol Molog they called it and the situation was even more magical than the archaic name implied. Within a hundred yards of the back door waved like sea-weed in the surge of the sun the lichen fringes of the dark hem of thick primaeval forest which belted this great mountain of fire and snow. When I knew it, it was still full of elephant, leopard, colobus, bushbuck, python and jumbo butterflies. Through the glass-panelled walls in front one looked down below on the Maasai plain, skimming away trembling, shimmering, flickering with haste and heat and flame of noonday sun, on into the blue in the direction of Somalia, as if it had no finality or horizon, since even what was a blue pencil circumference of vision elsewhere there was made of such space and light and immensities that blue of land and sky merged as one, and the last line of division was erased as in some dream vision of world without end.

There, while Michael flew five days a week to doctor where no doctors had been before and travelled the world in between to keep his unique service alive and expand it in accordance with the terrible medical necessities he increasingly uncovered in this vast area, Sue grew corn successfully, and following the seasons they harvested wheat twice a year. And how apt and with what poetic justice that it should have been corn she chose to grow. The difficulties of climate, parasites, disease, not to mention even the human, social and political ones that stood between Sue and her achievement, were almost insuperable. It always looked easy and beautiful enough to disguise the grim battle that made Ol Molog what it was, for one would land there with Michael on a Friday evening, within an hour of leaving Nairobi, right in the middle of fields of wheat which stood thick and high over us with tassels of pure gold between the aircraft and the level evening sun. But being from the land myself, I knew from regular visits over the years the heroic struggle that daily went into the making of it and marvelled at this wonder. Then, just when it was at its most beautiful and productive, the house was destroyed by fire. However, it was rebuilt and put into full production again. But at that moment the Tanzanian Government forced the Woods to 'sell the farm to the state' and they had to leave.

I myself would have found this last blow harder to take than destruction by fire. Yet I have never known either of them complain or utter one bitter, reproachful word over what was, making full allowance for all the ideological euphemisms advanced for the deed, an ungrateful and heartless eviction and more sinister still, an indication of the reappearance, although powerfully in reverse, of the same old arch-enemy of ours : racialism and colour prejudice. But they did not see it like this at all and found it so natural and just that far from being tempted into cutting their bond with Africa, they returned to the Kenya of their beginnings where Sue calmly, and with a touch surer than ever, made a new home for them.

She made it in a suburb of Nairobi called Karen. It was on the land that had once been part of Karen Blixen's estate, hard by the blue Ngong hills all readers of *Out of Africa* will remember. They made it not far from where Denys Finch-Hatton, who was the love of Karen's life, is buried, and where I used for years to go regularly on my beat up and down Africa, to put flowers on his grave at Karen's bequest. It is poetically just that *Go An Extra Mile* should have been written at Karen because all her suffering in the cause of what seemed so unlikely a love has found substance and increase in the life and work described in this book.

The main proof of this among the many others in the book is, of course, the African Medical and Research Foundation, which I knew when it was just a first-light glimmer in Michael Wood's eye. Today it is at last firmly established, still growing and a force of immense power for giving Eastern Africa the freedom from disease and want it needs to achieve a new freedom of mind and spirit for society. More, in the course of establishing such a Foundation, Michael Wood has rediscovered how dangerously sterile and self-defeating is the increasingly compartmentalized and impersonal approach to medical practice in the world. Both by deed and example he redirects medicine to the ancient and classical values which once made it so great an instrument of healing in the original meaning of the word, rooted in a common derivation wherein healing, holy and making whole, are one, and all essentials of the physician's art – a vocation which is complete only if its approach is as religious as it is scientific.

One of the outstanding by-products of his story indeed is that it has provided him with a means for making statements on medicine, missionaries, government, welfare services, religion and affairs that have a relevance far beyond Africa, and an immediacy greater for our own failing institutions and sick societies.

He has been enabled to do so because all he writes comes out of living and lived experience. Indeed, one of the main reasons why this straightforward account achieves so great an authority and dignity is because it never strays beyond the writer's own experience.

There remains only the necessity for a personal word about the Woods because they, as people, appear in these pages on the whole only indirectly and obliquely, by implication of what they have done. Their own personalities are, as it were, rationed in the discipline and necessities of the multiple and unremitting endeavour of their lives. As a result I feel compelled to speak, as they would not, of their generous and chivalrous human reality and to stress that they both are among the least angular and most varied yet rounded of friends I have ever had. All the variety and circumference however are, as far as Michael is concerned, centred in the fact that he is above all a born healer.

Archie McIndoe, who was in at the beginning of the Flying Doctor Service, once said to me that Michael was one of the most inspired surgeons he had ever met. But in a sense even the testimony of so great and expert a healer as McIndoe was irrelevant because I had over the years enough evidence of my own to substantiate the claim. All was implicit for me in a remark Michael made to me once after we had been listening to a piece of music in their room at Ol Molog. It was music wherein fateful tension and conflict of spirit were resolved in an immense Aeschylean acceptance and when the last chord of the cathartic conclusion had died away, Michael said, more to himself than to me, 'It is odd, but I never feel so calm and resolved myself, even now, as I do when I am in the middle of a truly serious operation.' Only someone who is speaking of the end for which he had been born, I believe, is capable of thought of that kind.

Besides, there was the more tangible evidence of ex-patients and one's own experience as well. I remember an occasion when Michael and Sue left me at the old Leopoldville, and flew on to Lambarene in the Gabon to see Albert Schweitzer. I saw them off at Brazzaville on the edge of the copper Congo one morning of a sun of burning sulphur. As they had to travel light in the primitive aircraft they left most of their luggage, including Michael's travelling surgical kit, behind with me.

At Lambarene Michael saw some truly horrific cases of elephantiasis. Talking to the nurses and doctors he was amazed to find that they did not know that elephantiasis could also be dealt with surgically. He mentioned this to Schweitzer at dinner the first night and offered to demonstrate how the relevant operation could be performed. Schweitzer accepted gratefully, but to Michael's horror he did not find a single instrument in the hospital surgery which he thought sharp enough for the operation. Undismayed by the fact that his own instruments were beyond reach or immediate summons, he did something which will surprise no one who reads the many illustrations of his gift for improvisation in this book. He always carried scores of Gillette blades with him. The next morning, with Sue to help, he performed the exceedingly complicated operation using in all, I think, seventy-six (the number seems riveted to my memory) razor blades, and Schweitzer and his staff were as grateful as they were enlightened.

Added to this, he is a born and inspired pilot. Indeed, this is an essential part of his remarkable achievement. Had not both Michael and Sue been truly modern and immediate in thinking and doing, the African Medical Research Foundation could never have become the great source of healing it is today. It was ultimately the fact that Michael's gift and vision of medicine was matched by his love of flying that produced recognition of the immense role the aeroplane could play medically in a country so vast, roadless, inhospitable and scattered as that part of Africa.

Not surprisingly, therefore, some of the most exciting things in this book are the accounts of Michael's medical missions by air over unmapped country with no external aids of communication. As reminiscences of pure adventure they are outstanding; wedded as they are to creative purposes of a life and death urgency, they are unique.

I have flown with him countless times all over Africa, with Sue as navigator, and once for days over impenetrable forests of the Congo and Central Africa in a single-engined aircraft. It was during one such flight over the Congo that I watched the cauli-flower world below open briefly, from time to time, to display its hidden wealth of rivers in a dazzle of sudden sun. They were of all colours. I remember green, blue, chocolate, chrome yellow, peacock, and Bible black. But after each brief revelation of water, the forest below would unfailingly close into its cauliflower cover again.

At the end of some four or five hours I could not help asking, 'Michael, if our engine gives out, what would you do?'

Without taking his eyes from his compass he said calmly, in the most everyday of voices, 'Oh, I'll just wrap the plane around a tree.'

This sounded as incomprehensible as lethal to me and I asked him what precisely he meant.

The explanation, he said, was quite simple. Some years before when Ernest Hemingway, on one of his hunting trips to Africa, had crashed in the bush and barely escaped with his life, an SOS had brought Michael flying to Hemingway's aid. After seeing to him (in a manner which Hemingway's widow subsequently told me impressed him so much that he remarked that if he ever needed surgical treatment again he would look for it not in New York but in Africa), Michael discussed the forced landing with the 'bush' pilot of Hemingway's plane. Michael was astounded that they could have survived it and asked the pilot, who had immense experience of flying over forest, desert and savannah, how he managed to achieve so miraculous a result.

'Oh,' the pilot said laconically, 'I just wrapped the plane around the nearest tree.'

I discovered then that this was an essential part of the bush pilot's art. When forced to land in forests or bush, he would aim the plane at the widest crack in the surface of the trees and try to hit the trunk of the most substantial tree available with the wing of his plane. The sideways impact would send the plane spinning like a top round the tree until its thrust was unwound and it sank, limp and bruised, to the ground.

On one occasion I flew with Michael and Sue in an ignorance

that was blissfully immune to any area of doubt, perturbed only because as the hours went by there was no sign of the mission landing ground for which we were heading. The sun went down and it began to darken quickly. I thought that we too would soon have to see how well our own plane could be 'wrapped round a tree'. I turned to look at Sue. The question in my mind must have been obvious from the expression on my face.

'Help Michael keep a look-out straight ahead as sharply as you can. By my reckoning we ought to see the landing ground at any minute now,' she said quickly.

And just before the bat-black minute close of the day, we saw the mission lights. In the last brown of the evening Michael put us safely down just before our supply of petrol ran out.

It is for me as if in this particular memory of a safe landing at nightfall, against all odds and appearances, in the Congo which inspired Conrad's *Heart of Darkness*, there is something of a metaphor of their lives: Sue the initiator and, out of her intuition of a freer and greater expression of human life on earth, inevitably the navigator in this story of transfiguration and translation from a European to an African idiom of life; Michael the doer and person born to give substance to the improbable intuition in the urgent here and now, and so pilot of an Africa that is not yet.

This then is the unique importance of this book. It shows how the bond between Africa and Europe is not only intact but also how, if the individual stands fast within all it evokes in him, as the Woods have done, it will live on. Perhaps finally it will do more than any combination of political and ideological forces can do to prevent a return to another round of the heart of darkness which increasingly threatens Africa, and to set it on the way of discovering a modern identity of its own.

LAURENS VAN DER POST
Africa, February 1978

Prologue:
A Maiden Flight

A sense of wonder is a virtue which seems to get lost as we leave childhood. Yet if we redevelop it and give it time it repays its dividends in human joy, awareness and a sense of belonging to the continuing miracle of life.

It springs from the standpoint of daring not to know and allowing the mind to revel in delights of appreciation without having to understand. Music can be appreciated and touch the heart strings without one having to know anything about crotchets and quavers. The enquiring human intellect seeks to know why, and when it knows why, something of the wonder is lost. Acceptance of life for what it is produces a calm, almost child-like, condition from which happiness can flow. It sometimes seems that the more we know the less we understand and the more miserable and haunted the quality of human life becomes.

For me, flying helped to redevelop my sense of wonder. The medium is indefinable in terms which really indicate its magical properties. Perhaps mountaineering conveys many of the same sensations. Standing on an alpine ridge and watching the clouds below or seeing the patchwork quilt of fields, forests and towns below comes close to conjuring up the same emotions and sensations. It is the cutting of the umbilical cord to mother earth which produces a new separate existence and an objectivity and detachment seldom realized when feet are on the level ground.

Flying has, too, a mystical quality. Air cannot be seen like water, and therefore its currents and movements are also invisible, as pilots know only too well and are at times painfully reminded of, in clear air turbulence. Experience gives a pilot a sixth sense of what to expect and as his knowledge of weather increases he begins to know in advance what he is likely to meet next. As the musician knows his notes and the poet his words, so the pilot must know the air in which he moves as the substance in which he must manipulate the control surfaces of his aircraft.

Unfortunately, flying in air-liners has largely removed this sense of close contact with the medium of air and it is only in light aircraft that a pilot can really feel the excitement and proximity of his medium. Again, air-liners fly so high that one is largely cut off from looking down on the earth and getting that intimate view which makes light-aircraft flying such a conscious pleasure. The same thing, of course, applies to large ocean-liners and small sailing-boats – the physical appreciation of the medium is reduced by the size of the vessel.

The machine is a tool; a means and not an end. The aeroplane is one of man's great inventions and a thing of great beauty. Almost more than any other factor it has revolutionized the lives of the last two generations. Only since the Second World War has transport by air been available on a large scale to the general public and perhaps this very fact has made us lose our sense of wonder, because it has become commonplace. One science which has greatly benefited from the aeroplane is medicine. The peaceful uses of aircraft are limitless but its application to the life of doctors showed me a new dimension and the possibilities of using this newfound tool to the benefit of humanity, especially in areas of the world where distances are large, roads are poor and infrequent, and medical men are few and far between. Early in my flying career the miracle of rapid transport was demonstrated to me in a way which had an indelible effect on my thinking.

I was reading peacefully at my home in Limuru, twenty miles outside Nairobi, one day in 1955, when the telephone rang and I was asked to fly to Lodwar, in the northern desert of Kenya, to see a man who had a head injury and needed urgent treatment. 'What is the story?' I asked. My informant, who worked in the Desert Locust Control Organization, said:

'We have had a radio message to say that one of our employees has had a head injury, is unconscious and requires evacuation to hospital.'

'All right,' I said. 'I should be with you by 2.00 p.m., with any luck.' I got my things together, drove down to Nairobi, picked up my medical bag and a stretcher and put them into the old Piper Tripacer which I shared at that time. As I hadn't been to Lodwar before, I worked out my course on the map and found I had to fly on a course of 350° for two hours and forty-five minutes if I could maintain a speed of 120 m.p.h. This was to be the first of many trips to Lodwar but then it was a novelty and I was flying over country I had never seen before. There were no navigational aids to help me, so I flew by dead reckoning and followed my route on the map. It was a fine day and the country was looking its best as I climbed back over Limuru and on above the Kinangop plateau along the western slopes of the Aberdare Mountains. Almost at once the medical problem faded from my mind and I concentrated on the business of flying. I made some calculations on paper about fuel consumption and the time I must leave Lodwar if I was to get back that day in daylight. The detachment from the earth below began to soothe me – no one could telephone me; no one could interrupt my thoughts. I was alone with my machine. I scanned the dials to check all was well. I listened to the engine which seemed to be making its accustomed sound and we sped on over Thompson's Falls and down into the Rift Valley. I could see the splurge of pink on the edges of Lake Hannington and I remembered that this was one of the favourite places for flamingoes in their thousands. Gradually the terrain changed and the earth became browner and sandier as the highlands were left behind and I approached the desert to the north. Leaving Lake Baringo just on my left, I came across some sharp peaks which rose to about 8000 feet. They were arid and treeless and there was no sign of life. The country of the Turkhana people stretched northward to the horizon and beyond, and my imagination began to play with the thought of what lives they led down below there. It must be a harsh struggle with the elements. What could they grow? How did they survive? Like all pastoral people they lived off their animals; milk and occasionally meat would be their spartan diet and so grazing would be their great worry and they would have to follow the rain. Every third year or so the rain would not be enough and people and cattle would die. It was a grim, relentless battle for survival, and viewed from above it was a marvel that anyone ever survived at all.

The wind is nearly always easterly in much of East Africa, so I knew I would probably have to allow 5° or so to maintain my correct track over the ground. I had been told that the best thing to do was to find the road around Lokichar and follow it in to Lodwar. The road was not very distinct when I found it but it seemed to be leading in the right direction so on I went into the desert, following the map and knowing I should hit the Turkwell river sooner or later as it crossed my course.

As I approached Lodwar, my mind changed gear again and I began to think of how I was going to transport this man to Nairobi if indeed he required to be. And then there was Lodwar – a typical white Beau Geste kind of town – over the river and down I came on to the large sandy strip. I parked up at the side of the strip where there was a lorry waiting to refuel me and got out feeling a little stiff. The temperature was around 100°F. and it hit me after the cool of Limuru. Down the track came two cars, the District Commissioner in one with some of his staff and the patient in the other driven by the sub-assistant surgeon with a medical orderly.

It was clear that they were all very disappointed about something and it was only inadvertently that I discovered that I had been expected to bring a nurse. These poor men had not seen a woman for months and I had robbed them of the chance. I never made that mistake again.

I enquired of these very smart, recently shaven, gentlemen what the details of the story were concerning the injured man, and the sub-assistant surgeon told me that the patient had been playing cards when his 'friend' had hit him between the eyes with a hammer. Everyone presumed that the patient had had one ace too many up his sleeve. This incident had occurred the evening before and the patient hadn't been conscious since. I found out what medical treatment he had been given and then undid the bandage on his head after he had been laid on my stretcher. The first thing I saw was brain under the dressings, so I hastily put them back in place. It was clear that the man was not deeply comatose and that he should be taken back to a reference hospital for X-rays and operative treatment. I asked that the patient should be given a sedative by injection and shortly afterwards this was done. We loaded our patient on his stretcher into the plane; no mean feat as the plane was small. His feet came over the co-pilot's seat in front while his head was at the back of the cabin. As fate would have it this proved to be a mistake.

Bidding my friends goodbye and after checking the aircraft I taxied out on to the strip again for take-off. It was 3.20 p.m. Soon I was heading back to Nairobi and my troubles seemed largely to be over. Little did I realize what was in store for me. After about an hour of travel and just when I felt that the sedative should have settled my patient nicely, I was alarmed to hear a groan and then the patient's left foot struck me a forceful blow on my right ear. I wished that I had arranged the man's head my end and that his feet had been the other. Clearly he was coming to from his coma and it looked as if I was in for an awkward fight to stop him disrupting the flying. I swore always to take a nurse in the future, a decision which I have never regretted. Fortunately I had the man strapped on his stretcher and about half an hour later the sedative really took over and he was quiet again.

As I approached the highlands to the south I saw what appeared to be a black curtain some forty miles ahead. It looked as if I was in for some weather problems. The next thing I saw was forked lightning and shortly afterwards the sky went dark and I was into rain. I had decided to go down low and see if I could keep the Rift Valley floor in sight and come out at Nakuru. Five minutes of being thrown round the sky was enough to convince me that I had better rethink my tactics. I did a 180° turn and went back the way I had come. I was happy about my fuel position but I knew I didn't have a lot of time to spare if I was to get into Wilson Airport before it was dark, as there were no night flying facilities at Wilson in those far-off days.

I decided to try and get south between the Aberdares and Mount Kenya, so I went eastwards to begin with across the Laikipia plains, hoping for a hole to get through around Rumuruti. I was thankful my patient remained quiet. The black curtain depressed me and I saw myself having to land on a small strip somewhere soon. I did not relish spending the night in the plane with a patient who might become obstreperous again, but more important I needed to get this patient to hospital as soon as possible. The agony was long and drawn out but somehow I managed to nose my way round the Aberdares, down by Nyeri station and over the foothills around Fort Hall and back to Wilson.

I learned a lot and frightened myself more than I care to admit. It was one of the first of many such bush flights. It was certainly good for my adrenalin secretion and I discovered a number of vital facts about flying in bad weather. Firstly, there is no substitute for what the airline pilots call 'route experience'. It is during the period of getting that experience that it behoves one to be very careful. As the old saying goes, 'There are many old pilots and many bold pilots but few who are old and bold.' Local knowledge is invaluable in bush flying and slowly one builds up a mental picture of what to expect, where the railway is, where there is a river or where there is a funny shaped hill. This mosaic of features gradually becomes one of the things which can automatically be recalled to mind and on which the bush pilot's life depends. Then, windscreen wipers are not fitted to small aircraft, which means you have to look out of the side window as the view ahead is obliterated in heavy rain. In this little plane there was a small triangular window which could be opened on the pilot's side and through it I could see the ground. Again, there is the vital question of when to turn round to escape putting one's neck into a noose. To do a 180° turn at the right time may be a life-saving decision. Never refuse to turn back if it is the wise thing to do. Then there is the local knowledge concerning the weather in each area of the country, the funk holes, and the alternative airstrips. Instinctively the pilot must accumulate all this information and be able to produce it when he most needs it as a conditioned reflex.

I landed at Wilson as it was getting dark and called for an ambulance to take my patient to what was then known as the King George VI Hospital. I drank a cup of coffee, left all thoughts of flying behind, and then went to the hospital with my patient. After getting him to bed in the ward I made a careful examination of his nervous system. He began to become restless again and reacted violently to any stimulus. X-rays showed he had a punched-out area of bone driven into the frontal area of his brain and this needed to be removed. I got him cleaned up, ordered some penicillin by injection and called the anaesthetist to see whether he was fit for operation. An hour later I had him in the operating theatre. It was not difficult to pick out the bone from the brain, wash the area out to remove infected débris and repair the damage. I was most worried about sepsis and leakage of the cerebro-spinal fluid, which acts as a buffer around the brain. When I had done what I could, I returned him to the ward with instructions to the nurses and left for home. I got in at 10.00 p.m., some twelve hours after I had left. The meal my wife gave to me was most welcome as I hadn't eaten since breakfast. Sunday is supposed to be a day of rest – on this occasion it was scarcely restful but full of interest and useful lessons had been learnt. Some six weeks later the patient was returned to Lodwar to his job, and as far as I know he is still playing cards, but with a scar on his forehead to remind him that it is better to lose a game than lose his life.

1
Africa

A friend of Susan's father came one day in 1946 to Queen's Elm Square in Chelsea where we were living and told us of a surgeon in Nairobi who badly needed an assistant to help him in his practice. After discussing this proposition for some time, we agreed to go for six months and see how we liked it.

Susan had not been back to Africa since the first year of her life when she had been carried in a hammock by her missionary parents from the Congo to the Nile. This amazing journey, which she described in her book *A Fly in Amber*[1], had always stuck in my imagination and I often used to think about it because it had a haunting quality. Her mother, Edith Buxton, had described to me the perils of that long safari and the dangers they had encountered before finally arriving at Juba and sailing down the Nile to Khartoum.

I remembered her description of Susan slung in a hammock dressed in a nappy and a topee and of how, during the journey, she had run out of milk for her tiny titian-haired daughter. This agonizing situation had played so much on her mind that when she finally arrived in Khartoum she went into the first shop and bought every tin of milk which she could see on the shelf as the relief of arriving in civilization again was so great.

[1] *A Fly in Amber*, Susan Wood, Harvill Press, 1964.

This habit must have clung to her because I remember during the war she sallied forth to the shops in Chelsea and came back home with a tea strainer which she claimed was the last in London. She finally collected thirteen tea strainers in this way which seemed to me a little excessive, but I understood where this collecting habit had originated.

I have always been so grateful to my mother-in-law who had taken me into her family as a down-at-heel medical student whom she must have felt was a poor match for her beautiful daughter. She has, over the years, been a very good friend and confidante and has, perhaps, been able to see my work in Africa as a continuation of her own and her husband's, though in a different field of endeavour. Her husband, Alfred Buxton, was killed in Church House by a bomb during the 1940 air raids, and it is one of the great regrets of my life that I never knew this remarkable pioneer, but I do know that Susan inherited many of his fine attributes which included a toughness of spirit, a love of Africa and a serene compassionate temperament. The story of Alfred Buxton has been told elsewhere[1] and also of the man he went to join in Africa, C. T. Studd[2], Edith's father. This grand old man, who started the World Evangelisation Crusade, had a remarkable life, which included playing cricket for England, becoming one of the 'Cambridge seven' in China and finally pioneering the new mission in the heart of Africa. The organization he started flourishes today and was the result of his uncompromising dedicated fundamentalist vision of Christianity and its task.

It took some time for us to find a passage to Africa in those days after the war when most of the ships were still troop carrying and the airlines were at an embryo stage of development. Eventually we were told that we had been allocated a cabin on a boat called the *Cairo*, which turned out to have been used by King Farouk as his private yacht and also by illegal immigrants on their way to Haifa. This vessel was due to set sail from Marseilles, to which we should have to travel overland via Paris. Thus started a nightmare journey which has so scarred my mind that I have never been able to contemplate a sea voyage from that day to this.

[1] *Alfred Buxton of Abyssinia and Congo*, Norman Grubb, Lutterworth Press, 1942.

[2] *C. T. Studd: Cricketer and Pioneer*, Norman Grubb, Lutterworth Press, 1973.

We had by then two children : Mark, aged two-and-a-half, and Janet, aged three months, and with all our paraphernalia we were seen off from Victoria station by our respective families just before Easter 1947. The excitement of packing and the very cold winter which we had endured had resulted in my asthma being at its worst, so I was not very good at heaving the luggage about. However, the journey as far as Paris was bearable, but from then on it deteriorated rapidly.

At the station in Paris we found there was a porters' strike and the seats in the train to Marseilles had been double booked. A free-for-all took place and somehow it was sorted out and we found ourselves jammed in our seats with Janet in a carry cot on the rack. The train wended its way southward through the night and the corridor was totally impassable with people sitting on their suitcases and blocking all passage to the lavatories. By this time my asthma was giving me a lot of trouble and Sue got out the adrenaline to give me a welcome jab in the arm. Clearly our fellow passengers thought I was a hard-line drug addict, but by then I was beyond caring.

The next problem to be solved was heating up Janet's milk. Sue tackled an almost impossible obstacle race down the corridor armed with a spirit lamp, milk, a bottle and Janet. It was a heroic struggle but somehow the water was boiled, Janet got fed and the nightmare journey continued. In the morning we eventually arrived at Marseilles, having experienced a modern version of the black hole of Calcutta. We were cramped, tired and cross with the effort of managing to survive but salvation appeared to be at hand.

I cannot remember how we finally got on board our 1300-ton steamer but I do remember the first glance at our cabin which was to be our home for the next three weeks. It was about six feet by four feet, smelt of fish and was dark and foreboding. Somehow we managed to get the children in and to rest and I then went on deck to see to the luggage. We had with us just what we could carry but the heavy luggage was supposed to be in a railway truck, which I soon discovered had been lost somewhere between Paris and Marseilles. We were told that the ship was due to depart shortly and a furious debate took place between the passengers, the purser and the porters on the quayside. Where was the luggage? The porters shook their shoulders and gesticulated in true Gallic style. I went to report this unwelcome news to Sue.

'But we can't start on this voyage without the children's things,' she said in her forthright manner.

'Right,' I said, 'we'll have to get off then if they don't appear.'

I hurried back on deck. Meanwhile it had become clear that our luggage had been found in some siding and that if we were prepared to hand over a sizeable amount of cash the porters would bring the luggage on board. Blackmail on these occasions always seems to work and we had no alternative but to give in. We suspected that the luggage had been hidden round the corner all the time and that this was simply a ruse to extract some easy money. By this time the passengers were fuming with righteous indignation and very apprehensive about the coming voyage. It transpired that there was a cosmopolitan crew, that we were flying the Panamanian flag and that the ship had never been out of the Mediterranean before – not good omens.

However, we settled down and the fresh sea air did us a lot of good after the closed compartment of the French train. We took stock of our surroundings and made friends with a dentist and his wife who proved to be very good value. We were the only medical people aboard, as we soon found out as the purser sought our aid for various ailing passengers. We unpacked and managed to get things straight in the cabin, though we anticipated major problems in the Red Sea from the heat. We were not disappointed.

Mark was at the age when his main interest in life was dashing to the side of the ship to look over. The rails were skimpy in the extreme and on occasion to prevent him feeding the sharks I had to throw myself in true rugger style to the ground and grab him by the ankle. Janet was less mobile and therefore less of a problem. As the voyage went on, we found a place up in the bows where we could leave her safely in her carry cot in the fresh air. Occasionally she was washed by a fine spray, which cooled her off during our passage through the Red Sea.

The main chores were washing the nappies and looking after Mark on deck. Sue and I tossed up. I favoured the nappies every time as the vigil with Mark on deck was too harrowing. I remembered the old story of King George V and his Chaplain when on a Sunday morning the King explained to his Chaplain that he had tossed up to see whether he should go to church or play golf, adding wryly that he had had to toss up eighteen times before he was able to go off to his golf. I felt the same about the nappies.

At Port Said we were able to disembark, and while wandering around the shops stretching our legs, an Egyptian came up to me and tried to sell me a grand piano! We laughed so much at this ridiculous suggestion that the man became quite embarrassed, but after all he had not seen our cabin or he might have enjoyed the joke a little more.

We survived through the Red Sea in appalling heat but we took mattresses up on deck and were just able to bear it in this way. We stopped at Aden, which gave us another chance to take a walk while the ship was being refuelled. We were then launched into the Indian Ocean. Two episodes still remain in my memory as we beat our way down the African Coast. The lesser concerns the first mate, who was caught misbehaving with a lady passenger and was clapped into irons and deposited in some deep dungeon in the bowels of the ship.

Of more serious consequence, we noticed that our ship was moving slower and slower through the water and at the same time the funnel was belching forth red-hot ashes which floated down on to the deck. Then suddenly the awning over the deck was on fire and a great blaze took place, with the passengers scurrying for safety. The fire was soon under control but the ship continued to slow down until it finally stopped. None of the passengers knew what had happened, but some time later it was given out that there was trouble with the boilers. The ship had no way on it and we were at the mercy of the sea, which fortunately was moderately calm. Then, to our relief, we discovered there were six ex-RNVR officers on board who offered their services to the Captain to diagnose the mechanical problem.

After the fire had been extinguished in the boilers and enough time had elapsed to allow them to cool off, it transpired that the engine had not been maintained since 1904 when it had been designed in Glasgow; certainly the pipes from the boiler carrying the steam were totally blocked. A kind of decarbonizing operation was launched and the pipes were cleaned through by our gallant RNVR officers. Finally, eighteen hours later, we got under way, again, much to everyone's relief.

One last final obstacle had to be overcome, namely finding Mombasa. Our captain, who had never been to Mombasa before, was duly instructed how to approach Mombasa harbour, a pilot

was taken aboard and finally we berthed amid scenes of unparalleled rejoicing. I swore that I would never set foot on a
boat again. From that moment on flying became a necessity and
although it was some years before I learnt to fly myself, the die
was cast.

Mombasa was a great adventure for us. It was the first time
I had been in Africa and after the *Cairo* everything appeared
especially inviting and intriguing.

The same evening we boarded the train for Nairobi and
were pleasantly surprised with the roomy carriages, comfortable
sleepers and excellent food. We slept from sheer exhaustion and
relief at leaving the ship, and in the morning had our first introduction to the Kenya countryside as we moved slowly across the
Athi plains towards Nairobi. Game abounded and we sat fascinated
at our first glimpse of this highland country while watching
giraffes, zebras and wildebeeste in profusion. I took a deep breath
of the alpine air and from that moment on my asthma was
largely controlled and has seldom worried me seriously since.

The house of my surgeon employer, Gerald Anderson, was in
Muthaiga, a suburb of Nairobi some four miles from the centre.
Caroline Anderson, although bed-ridden with paralysis, welcomed
us and made us feel at home at once. Gerald was busy with his
practice and we did not meet him till later in the day. The
Andersons had arranged for us to stay in a bamboo cottage at
the bottom of their garden. This was cosy and comfortable and
we revelled in the freedom to move around after our cramped
quarters aboard the infamous *Cairo*.

Looking back on those early days I suppose, like most other
visitors to Nairobi, we were quickly enthralled by the scene. The
gardens were beautiful and the flowering shrubs and trees a
constant joy. The climate is, perhaps, the best in the world, with
warm days and cool nights and sun most of the year round. It was
bliss for the children to be able to run out of doors without having
to dress up in coats, scarves and other encumbrances.

I found in Gerald Anderson a delightful colleague who had
been in Africa since he was six and who was really part of the
scene. He was not only a highly competent surgeon but also a very
knowledgeable physician as well. In the days when he started to
practise he had had to be a jack-of-all-trades. Nevertheless, his
academic record was remarkable and he even took his Mastership

in surgery during his forties. With a strong Christian conviction and compassion he set a very high standard and I was very fortunate to have my surgical introduction to Africa with him to lean on. He was most generous in giving me a start and I learnt a great deal from him, not only about surgery but about dealing with patients.

Two weeks after our arrival Sue woke up with a splitting headache and I rushed up the garden to seek Gerald's advice. Within a few hours it was shown that she had meningitis. I took her lying down in my car to the Infectious Diseases Hospital – an *ayah* was found for the children and the next few weeks proved an anxious time for us all. I was trying to get going in the practice, keep an eye on the children and be with Sue every spare minute.

The infection was probably caught aboard the *Cairo*, as two other passengers succumbed to the same illness. Sue was the only one to survive. Her life was saved by the devotion of a nursing sister, Eileen Cook, who became a close friend and later married Geoffrey Timms, another stalwart friend and a well-known pathologist in Nairobi. I have always felt an enormous debt of gratitude to Eileen whose skill, patience and devotion made the whole difference to Sue while she was struggling to hold her own against the infection. Slowly she pulled through, the danger passed and life became bearable again, as I could reassure Sue's mother that she was recovering and would soon be up and about.

When I was struck down with a serious illness many years later, I remember being particularly impressed again with my nurses. I have always felt that all doctors should be really ill occasionally because then they learn to appreciate their nursing staff. It is quite different to be in the sick bed rather than at the bedside. Nursing, until recently, has been a strangely unemancipated profession with long hours, poor pay and often heavy work. Fortunately, now, conditions are much better. African girls have taken to nursing like ducks to water. They are usually quiet, have good hands and a real concern for their patients. Initiative is perhaps lacking in some of them but their even temper and willingness easily make up for this lack. Doctors probably see their patients for a few minutes a day but the nurses are with them all the time and are often the best judges of how a particular patient is progressing.

Sue recovered and got back her strength on the shores of Lake Naivasha. Friends at Naivasha treated Sue like another daughter and I loved the weekends I was able to take up there as they gave me my first insight into the pleasures and problems of settler life. From those days onwards I always wanted to farm myself and this was to be an ambition which later we were able to realize. There is something unique about farming at 5000 feet on the equator. It is perhaps difficult to define and it is this indefinable character of the life which is so intriguing. It must be a combination of factors which makes the life so idyllic, challenging and yet at times immensely frustrating. It is easy to enumerate the obvious favourable items such as the climate, the breathtaking scenery, the warmth of the sun by day, the cool evenings with a log fire, the challenge of developing new land, the friendliness of the African and so on. But this does not wholly explain the enchantment, and only experiencing it all can really convince one of the particular joy of farming in Africa.

It is often said by those with a cynical turn of mind that the longer you live in Africa the less you understand it. Unfortunately there is a considerable grain of truth in this paradox. The more you know the more baffled you become; or so it seems.

This was still in the colonial days and scarcely anyone realized how short they were going to be. Sue and I felt instinctively that it was vital to move into the era of independence while there was still a modicum of goodwill left. We feel that the view was justified particularly if one considers the predicament in which Rhodesia finds itself today. Kenya managed to come through the sound barrier remarkably unscathed despite a rebellion and other hazards along its path. And now, fourteen years after independence, a great deal has been accomplished and Kenya can claim to have created as viable a multi-racial state as anywhere in Africa. That may not be saying much and no one could claim that it is anywhere near perfect.

On the medical side I derived great satisfaction in helping to get the blood transfusion service going and joining with a small band of like-minded citizens to develop our hospitals and build new ones. One amusing incident took place at this time. I became involved in the Red Cross and was Director of the Kenya Branch for about five years. During this period I was able to start a Flying Ambulance Service which was the precursor of the Flying Doctor

Service. We hired a plane for special emergency cases and gained some experience in the various pitfalls which bedevil this type of enterprise. The Duke and Duchess of Gloucester were paying a formal visit to Kenya and I was asked to bring the Red Cross Ambulance plane to Eastleigh Airport to be inspected by their Royal Highnesses just before they departed for the United Kingdom. We had some difficulty with the plane, as one side of the undercarriage gave trouble that morning, which left the port wing drooping nearly to the ground, and there was only half an hour to go before we were due to be on parade. I clambered into my uniform which somehow seemed an incongruous cross between that of a field marshal and a cinema commissionaire. Anyhow, I remember feeling particularly foolish in it. At the last moment the plane was fixed and we flew over to Eastleigh, which was only three or four minutes' flight. Susan was laid out on a stretcher and loaded into the plane and I shoved the prettiest nurse I could find into a seat beside her. When the royal party arrived I took them over to the Red Cross plane and explained how we operated the ambulance service. The Duchess went forward and through the door of the aircraft addressed the pretty nurse.

'How many times have you been up in the ambulance plane?' she asked.

'Never,' said my dumb blonde.

In looking back on those early days I remember that there never seemed to be enough time to accomplish all the things that were waiting to be done. We had two more children, Hugo and Katrina; we went to farm in Limuru and built a house there; helped to run the Capricorn Africa Society, and Susan even ventured into the field of politics, standing for parliament on a liberal ticket. We all knew she did not stand a chance because this election was run on a communal roll and only Europeans could vote on it. What were considered then dangerously liberal ideas would be stamped as downright reactionary today. We thought of a brilliant slogan, 'Put ginger into Nairobi North', which played up Sue's red hair. She got only 17 per cent of the votes but we enjoyed the campaign enormously. She is a very good public speaker and it gave her a chance to say things which we felt needed to be said at that time. It has been some small compensation to know that many of the things she advocated have since become reality.

It is very easy to get involved in Africa because there is so much to do. Susan and I found that although we had come out for only six months in the first place, we never really thought of going back to London. I was busy with my surgical practice and Susan was kept busy by the children, but we also enjoyed building the house at Limuru and starting to farm a hundred and fifty acres.

Making the garden was a delight as everything grows so quickly in Africa and Susan had a natural eye for it. She has made a number of gardens in Africa now, and each one has reflected her sense of design and colour. My contribution has been minimal but I always had a great feeling of rest and composure when going round the garden and seeing how everything was doing. Susan had known instinctively that she had to build a secure base for the children, and for me to return to from my peripatetic wanderings. She did it without any fuss as she is a natural nest-builder. The children perhaps never realized the care she lavished on them because they had never known anything different.

In an amateur way we ran a lovely herd of jerseys, which gave me enormous pleasure, and we were gradually introduced into the art of farming by a splendid Kikuyu cowman called Gageche, who taught us a great deal and saved us from making too many errors. We kept battery chickens, grew onions and tried a number of experiments. My limited tasks in all this enterprise were restricted to what could be termed the surgical aspects. Two incidents stand out in my memory, both of which caused a marked degree of psychological trauma.

We had two jersey bulls and the larger one was quite a handful. It was decided as he grew bigger that he must have a ring in his nose to control him, and I was detailed to perform this cosmetic operation. We had great difficulty in coaxing the bull into the fenced entrance to the cattle dip, but finally, by using guile in the form of a dainty heifer, we were able to persuade the bull to enter the pen. A major effort then ensued to secure him by placing poles in front and behind him and by tying his legs to the tough cedar uprights of the crush. A rope was put round his horns and by pulling hard we secured his head to a post. There was much heaving and grunting and at any minute we felt the bull might get loose.

I had been hanging about in the background in a cowardly

fashion while this performance went on, encouraging everyone else, but now there was no excuse for me to shirk my duty so I advanced with the weapon in hand. The ring was made so that it could hinge open, revealing a sharp-pointed piece of metal which had to be pushed through the cartilage of the septum of his nose. There was then a small screw which had to be inserted after the ring was closed so that it did not come undone again.

With unparalleled skill I managed to get the sharp point through the right place in the nose, though looking into the eye of the bull from close quarters it appeared to me that he was not overpleased. He snorted and heaved but the ropes held him. I closed the ring, got out the small screw and a screwdriver and prepared to complete the operation. At this moment the bull gave an extra heave and in my fright I dropped the screw in the long grass. I could not find it anywhere. A quick consultation took place and we saw that the only hope was to catch the other bull, who was more manageable, take out the ring from his nose, and substitute it into the nose of the large bull. This was finally accomplished and the big bull could be loosed, as we now had a bull-stick through the ring and he was under control. I was led away shaking from my ordeal and thanking my lucky stars that I had not trained as a vet. The family never let me forget this performance.

On another occasion, I was given the rather macabre task of despatching a cow. I cannot remember whether the animal was ill or whether we needed some meat, but I tethered the poor animal to a tree and was determined to make a clean job of it. I shot it between the eyes at close range with a .22 rifle. It merely shook its head as if it had a mild headache.

'Release the rope and let the cow fall,' I said confidently. As soon as the rope was removed, instead of falling over dead as I had expected, the animal took off at a quick gallop and did two circuits round the farm, followed by a motley crowd of farm-hands who tried to corner her. It is easy to imagine my chagrin. Gageche laughed till he cried, rolling on his back in paroxysms of mirth. I was never called in in this capacity again. The wretched animal was finally caught and despatched, but my authority and confidence never really recovered.

Life went on at a busy pace and I found myself helping to build hospitals and becoming Director of the Kenya Red Cross, while

Susan continued to undertake a mass of new things as well as bringing up the children.

It was at about this time that I decided to put some of my ideas into practice and learn to fly. Every evening after work I went to the small civil aerodrome on the outskirts of Nairobi and clambered into a Piper Cub, sharing the controls with a redoubtable instructor. I would head north for Limuru and fly over our house, high above the highlands, busy with the controls and unconscious of the applause of the family on the ground.

I found flying relatively straightforward and much akin to sailing, which had been an early sport of mine.

The discipline of flying, with its emphasis on checking every detail, intrigued me and the mental concentration required, on which safety depends, added a certain spice to the whole venture. Pilot error is the commonest cause of accidents and all the time there is a conscious effort to eliminate the blunders to which the human being is prone. Slowly I learnt from my mistakes, and from those made by other pilots. However, there seems no end to the possibilities for error and it is this thought which keeps a pilot in constant preparedness for the next unpredictable occurrence.

2
Surgeon

My overriding ambition as a small boy was to drive a taxi with yellow wheels. I remember thinking that this would be the ultimate joy and that nothing else was really worth considering. Perhaps unfortunately my views changed as I grew older and after battling with asthma for many years, which caused many setbacks in my undistinguished school career, I finally went into medicine, after nearly three years in architecture first. My patient father, before allowing me to change to a medical career, sent me to an institution where I was interviewed and examined to determine to what career I was suited. I remember having to write an essay on the civil service in ten minutes, do a whole lot of progressive matrices and mental arithmetic, and be grilled by my interviewer who attempted to assess my limited abilities. After about four hours I left this scene of torture and quickly forgot about it. However, some two weeks later my father received a bulky manuscript which set out the results and made some recommendations. I was to be an estate agent, was the remarkable conclusion. Apparently it was thought that I was good with people but quite unsuited to a medical career, as this would be too long and arduous for me. My father must have breathed a sigh of relief as he thought he was saved from the expenses of another long training; but the report finally and irrevocably made up my mind that I would do medicine come what may. I would show them what I was made of. I remember reading a brochure put out by this organization which advised on careers. There was something nauseatingly smug about it. One of the letters in it read something like this:

Dear Sir,

Twenty-one years ago you recommended that I should join the Sudan police. I thought, therefore, you would be interested and pleased to know that I accepted your advice and have enjoyed a most successful career. I have recently been appointed Commissioner of Police.

Yours faithfully,

My father gave in graciously and allowed me to switch careers. When I finally passed my specialist exams in surgery many years later, after numerous trials and tribulations, I reminded my father of the old report which had advised me to be an estate agent. I had, in my mind, written a letter to the careers organization which ran:

Dear Sir,

Some fifteen years ago I was advised by your organization to become an estate agent and forget all ideas of embarking on a medical career. I thought you would be interested to know that I ignored your advice and have since qualified as a specialist in surgery. I am most grateful to you for helping me to make up my mind to do what I always wanted.

Yours faithfully,

Michael Wood.

Of course this would have been childish and grossly unfair and I am sure I have largely misrepresented the situation. However, it remains in my mind as the time when the die was cast, and I have never regretted it.

I struggled through medical school at the Middlesex Hospital in London and enjoyed it all immensely, though the war started soon after and our school was moved first to Bristol and then Leeds during the time of the so-called 'phoney' war before the Blitz began. We returned to London and experienced the bombing during its various stages. I became inured to the disturbances, managed to concentrate on the text books and take a never-ending stream of exams. It never crossed my mind that Britain could be defeated, though, looking back on this time, it really was a miracle that we survived those early days and that the Battle of Britain was won by a very narrow margin. Perhaps it was the last time that amateurism got by without being patronized by the professionals. Within the British people there emerged an amazing stoicism, a refusal to contemplate defeat and a wonderful camaraderie, the like of which has sadly never been seen since. Britain has always had the reputation of not waking up till the last moment. Again today it is perilously late for her to come to terms with reality. Only recently Alexander Solzhenitsyn has felt compelled to utter what he feels to be the truth and this did shock the country with some realization of its predicament. The melancholy descent into bureaucratic boredom, economic insolvency and the tyranny of the unions has brought Britain once again to a crisis in its history. I still believe that she will take heed at this the eleventh hour and we shall see again a flowering and renaissance of the talents which have lain dormant for three decades. If this is a wrong diagnosis, the world will be a poorer place.

My war service was short and unmemorable but when I was qualified as a doctor I was able to make a small contribution in dealing with the bomb casualties and the wounded members of the armed forces who were evacuated to Britain. Something has to progress in wartime and surely surgery is one of the main beneficiaries. The coming of penicillin made a huge difference to the treatment of war wounds and the recovery rates became much quicker.

Like so many others whose job involved staying at home, I became accustomed to the scream of bombs and almost blasé about them. I was lifted off my feet in the King's Road, blown from my bed by a V1 'buzz bomb' and on one occasion had the experience of believing that another buzz bomb was about to hit me between the eyes as it came up Berners Street at rooftop height, when I was fire-watching on the roof of the hospital. The wing tipped a roof and the machine fell into Greek Street, causing some two hundred and fifty casualties who were shortly brought into the hospital and kept us all busy for a long time. One became fatalistic as a result of repeated near-misses, and the Middlesex Hospital was particularly fortunate in emerging almost unscathed from the onslaught.

At the weekends, I used to get down to my parents' house in South Oxfordshire and I remember well my duties in the Home

Guard. Today it is scarcely credible to think that our patrol had only one ·303 rifle and no ammunition. If a German paratrooper was sighted we were instructed to bicycle up to the schoolmaster's house and get five rounds of ammunition which were locked up in the school safe. Pikes and staves were issued but fortunately we were never called upon to wield them. I somehow feel that our encounter with German paratroopers would have been rather one-sided.

The surgery of war wounds is useful apprenticeship for the young surgeon but no one in their senses would wish to spend their time dealing with the hideous mutilations which modern weaponry produces. There is a new battlefront today which is waged on the roads and the appalling loss of life never seems quite to register with the public. I believe it is true to say that more lives have been lost on the roads in the USA than in all the wars put together since the beginning of the twentieth century involving American soldiers. This is but one of the hundreds of statistics which are bandied about today, but somehow they do not appear to get through. Accidents between the ages of 18 and 25 in men are the single commonest cause of death in most of the industrialized countries.

Coming nearer home, there can be few people today who do not know of close relatives or friends who have been killed or injured in this modern form of war. It touches us all and perhaps surgeons are more aware of this tragedy than anyone else as they know that their hospital beds are full to overflowing with this type of casualty.

One example must suffice to illustrate what this new scourge means today and what skills have to be brought to bear to try and limit the ravages of the road.

Surgery is a mixture of many skills, of science, of art and of manual dexterity. The technical side of surgery can be learnt with practice like any other technique. Speed can be learnt, though it is not an essential quality. There is the nice story which describes three categories of surgeons: one type, the master surgeon, makes all operations look easy; the second type, the average surgeon, makes the difficult operations look difficult and the easy operations look easy; while the third type manages to make even the easy operations look difficult! It is the task of most of us to try and escape from the third category.

Apart from the obvious attributes with which a surgeon must attempt to equip himself, there are other more subtle skills which have to be learnt by experience. Surgical judgement is the virtue which we all try to nurture; the quality made up of a series of indefinable, intuitive particles. I worked for a time with a surgeon who had acquired this virtue to an uncanny degree. Although unable to impart his knowledge verbally because he was strangely inarticulate, he could, nevertheless, by example, instil in his students some of the magic which he held at his finger-tips. He knew the answers but could not tell you why he knew them. He could teach but only by demonstration. The combination of eye, touch, memory and other unnamed sources of instruction is more important to a surgeon than either straight manual dexterity or erudite scientific knowledge, though clearly he needs these as well. He has to develop X-ray eyes which enable him to peel back mentally the layers of tissue and divine what is taking place in the depths of the human body. Only experience can help him develop and recall similar situations and conditions which finally place the pieces of the jig-saw puzzle in their correct position, thus revealing a clear picture.

What is it that we call 'touch' in a particular pianist? What special attribute does he possess which enables him to make a note sound in a certain way? Can we define it? I do not believe we can. And so it is with a surgeon's touch, the mystery which defies adequate description and for which words are not available. It is unique and compassionate, gentle yet strong.

Can there be an emanation from him who touches to the touched? A difference of electrical potential, a type of wave as yet unknown to science? Such a tactile vibration transmitted from one human being to another or to a note or canvas might help explain the different qualities in what we call 'touch'. Extra-sensory perception is a well-recognized phenomenon and yet do we know the path of transmission? It is comforting then to dwell on subjects of human ignorance and to realize that our knowledge is still crude and small in comparison with the total knowledge incorporated in our universe. It makes us humble and that is another essential virtue for the surgeon.

A young girl aged twenty, whose family was known to me, was involved in this battlefield on the roads when returning from the cinema in the evening with her fiancé. I was called at 11.45 p.m.

when I was sleeping soundly. I had gone to bed early because I was flying early the next morning to operate three hundred miles away. It was the mother who called me and she was so distressed it was difficult for me to assess really what had happened. I dressed and drove into the hospital and was met by the parents and the fiancé. Apparently they had had an encounter with a lorry which had been on the wrong side of the road. To avoid the lorry he had left the road and hit a tree at about forty m.p.h. The girl sitting by his side had been thrown through the windscreen. He had held on to the steering wheel and though he had a bruised chest he was not seriously injured. This accident had happened only an hour before. I left to see the girl and promised to come back and tell them what needed to be done. Talking to relations is never easy when a life hangs in the balance but I have found that most people appreciate the truth and like to know what is happening. There is no place for deceit or prevarication. It is not your life and you have no right to hide the truth. It can be imparted with tact and compassion but anything less than the truth builds up problems for the days ahead.

Up in the ward the house surgeon had been busy treating the girl for shock and blood loss. The laboratory results were expected shortly but in the meantime an intravenous infusion was being given and the nurses had cleaned up the patient, dressed her in hospital nightclothes and administered a sedative to calm her. She had been concussed and dazed but was now conscious.

The ward was quiet and all the lights out except the one over the girl's head. Curtains had been pulled around the bed and as I parted them I saw a nurse by the bedside taking the blood pressure. I stood and waited as the nurse finished her job and wrote her findings on the chart. We did not need to speak. The nurse's expression conveyed her concern and understanding of the seriousness of the case, and I was encouraged by her clean, neat, professional appearance. I thought of the times when I had been ill myself and how grateful I had been for the nurses who are really in the front line when it comes to a patient's comfort. They see the patients all the time whereas the doctor comes and goes and only sees the patients for maybe a few minutes in the day. I approached the bed and signed to the nurse to help me remove the bandages which had been put on in the casualty department. They were blood-stained and covered almost all of her head and neck except for a few tufts of hair which protruded through them, and immediately reminded me of what she looked like when I had last seen her. She had long dark hair, brown eyes, a generous mouth and an intriguing expression.

When I lifted the bandages I was horrified by what I saw. Any surgeon is used to seeing unpleasant sights but it is always worse when you know the person involved. I held her wrist to feel her pulse which was rapid but of good volume. I lent towards her and called her name. There was some response but no real recognition. Her face had been so severely damaged that her voice was impaired and what she said made no real sense to me. She was still having what amounted to a nightmare and she was frightened, in pain, and did not know where she was.

In undertaking my examination I did not want to hurt her more than was absolutely necessary. I started at the top of her head where there were a number of long lacerations – the blood had clotted. Her forehead had been lifted in one large flap of tissue from the eyebrows to her hair margin. Her eyes were undamaged but the lids terribly swollen and torn. Her nose was broken and she had fractures of both her upper and lower jaws. There were multiple smaller lacerations of her cheeks and chin and a long deep cut across her neck which was still bleeding. The rest of her was largely undamaged apart from a broken wrist. Her face had taken the main impact. As the car had decelerated she was thrown forward and her forehead had gone through the windscreen followed by the rest of her body. I had to get some X-rays taken, arrange for the theatre to be prepared, find an anaesthetist, see the relatives again and see that my instruments were ready.

The house surgeon dealt with the X-ray department and asked the duty anaesthetist if he could start the case at 1.30 a.m. Sorrowfully I went downstairs to talk to the relatives. I sat them down in the sister's office, arranged a cup of tea for them and then told them what I had found. I did not spare them the seriousness of the injuries and I outlined what I intended to do. They took it all remarkably well. At least they knew what they had to face.

We started to put the blood in by transfusion and I went to look at the X-rays. She had five fractures of the facial bones which would require wiring to restore the normal anatomical position and hold the bones until they healed.

There is one compensation for operating at night: the hospital is quiet, telephone calls infrequent, and there is less hurry. The theatre staff arrived looking bleary-eyed from sleep and soon everything was ready. Our patient was wheeled from the ward and I had a short word in her ear which probably did not really register.

I went off to scrub up as the anaesthetist gave her the first injection and she passed into total unconsciousness. To me this is always an important moment because you know your patient is out of pain and psychologically you no longer have to think of their personality as a human being. It is temporarily switched off and you are left to get on with the job uncluttered by the emotions of another mind. You know, too, that you will soon be back with your patient's conscious feelings and that this is only a brief interlude.

I thought of the immense advances in anaesthesia and how it has become one of the great boons of the twentieth century. We take it for granted now but it is a merciful skill which puts the patient into suspended animation and anonymity.

The ritual of the operating theatre had begun: the scrubbing up, the clatter of bowls and instruments, the gowns, caps and masks and the powerful lights all set the stage for the opening scene. During this time I began to concentrate my mind on the technical problems and talked to the theatre sister about the instruments I wanted, the sutures and the rest of the paraphernalia of a theatre, the sucker, the diathermy machine, the spotlight. Finally I discussed the position of the patient and whether it was possible to sit down because I knew it was going to be a long session. All the dressings were taken off and the skin carefully cleaned with an antiseptic solution. We then put on the sterile towels until the whole table was covered. The lights were focused and we could begin. A detailed look at the wounds confirmed the seriousness of the injuries. I decided to deal with the neck wounds first. This must have been the result of a jagged piece of glass cutting the neck as she went through the windscreen. The muscles which were partly severed had protected the vital structures such as the carotid arteries and the larynx. I removed some road dirt, irrigated the wound and started to sew up the layers.

'4/0 catgut, please, Sister, on an atraumatic needle.'

'Plain or chronic, sir?' she answers.

'Plain, please.'

'Give me the small needle holder.' She hands it to me. Approximating the torn tissue is a painstaking job but there is no real difficulty. Finally the skin is brought together with very fine nylon and I am ready to tackle the face.

The human face expresses so much of the personality behind it. The expressions of the face are legion and each line tells a story. To resculpture a face by surgery is a work of art – perfection is never reached after severe injury, but the essential is to get as close as possible and therefore to restore and heal the personality behind the features and their expression.

Firstly the bone structure must be put together because on this framework are draped the muscles of expression and the skin. If the floor of the orbit is at a different level on each side by even a millimetre, the symmetry of the face is destroyed and the level of the eyes affected. And so I set to work to expose the fracture sites, approximate them to their correct anatomical position and wire them together. This is done by making small holes on each side of the fracture and passing stainless steel wire through them and pulling the bone together. This took time but was eventually accomplished. The teeth were wired together so that the jaws splinted each other in the correct position of the bite. The final fixation of the wires of the jaws is left to the end of the operation so that the anaesthetist can get to the back of the throat where secretions and blood are sucked out.

Fortunately the facial nerves which supply most of the muscles of expression were intact. This gave me encouragement that the final expression could be restored. Patiently the muscles were sutured with fine catgut and the small vessels were picked up and their ends coagulated with the diathermy machine. Finally came the moment to restore the skin. The saying, 'Beauty is only skin deep,' is, like most such things, only a half-truth. In fact beauty is the aggregate of many factors, some of which are more sensed than seen. There is the classical form of a model face which may be accepted as near perfection, but we all know that real beauty is less definable and appears with other ingredients of a more spiritual or mystical nature. Complexion, colour, form, contour and proportion all add to this quality which we loosely call beauty, but expression is perhaps the most telling ingredient of them all. A face which is beautiful in form can be ruined by a sour expression, or can look mask-like and lifeless if not imbued with animation. We talk about a warm expression – what is it that constitutes warmth in a face? This is one of the riddles of life which has teased artists through the ages. The smile of the Mona Lisa has that bewitching, intriguing quality which adds such an air of mystery and instantly sets up a questioning curiosity in the mind of the beholder. What is she thinking? What was she really like? What secrets does she hold? Beauty is a complex concept which does not simply depend on skin.

I go on bringing the structures together until the subcutaneous layer has been sewn and only the skin is left. Scars are the story which the patient reads afterwards. How can we camouflage them or disguise them? Certain tricks of the trade are helpful. I try to break up the scars so they do not run in one long line. I hide them in the lines of expression wherever possible. I sew the skin with the very finest of sutures to minimize the stitch marks. Some scars are easier to hide than others; scars on the convexities of the face are going to receive more light; scars under the jaw are in shadow and less visible. It is 5.00 a.m. as the last stitch goes in; the concentration breaks as I straighten up and begin to be conscious that my back is aching. My eyes are weary and my bed seems to be beckoning me. I clean up around the wounds, take a final long look at the human canvas on which I have been working for over three hours and pass the patient over to the gentle care of the nurses.

There are several more jobs to do before I can leave the hospital. I must write up the post-operative orders in the notes, being particularly careful to instruct the nursing staff what to do if the patient is sick with her jaws wired together. What will she need in the way of sedatives and pain-killers? And then, while changing, I begin to think what can I say to the relatives who have had such a long vigil outside. They won't understand that the face is going to look bruised and swollen for some time. For the surgeon, who has seen these things many times before, there are comforting thoughts as he knows the amazing recuperative powers of nature, particularly in the young. How can he persuade the relations that his handywork must not be judged for some weeks to come?

With these thoughts chasing through my mind, I brace myself

for one more ordeal with the patient's mother. Can I summon up the compassion and the understanding and convey it across the distance which separates one human being from another? At least I can try. I see the mother's tear-stained face. I sense all the love which has gone into the bringing up of this girl, and now this tragedy, this disappointment. I hear myself trying to tell her what I have tried to do. I put my hand on her shoulder as I know the comfort that human touch can bring. I persuade her to go home and rest and try and forget for a little while, and I will come and see her again in the evening. Then there is the fiancé to talk to – how can I help to assuage his sense of guilt? He will have to live with the knowledge that at least he was partly responsible for this tragedy. He will have to look at this injured face which he has loved, fondled and kissed, and his love will be severely tested over the coming weeks. He will have to look at her eyes through her swollen lids and comfort her with his care and devotion. It will not be easy. I tell him what it will entail – there is no point in prevaricating – I am not going to promise miracles because I am not a miracle worker. There is no magic wand in my hand.

There is really no point in going to bed but I get home and have a bath before going to the airport. I am due to fly at 7.00 a.m. During the war as a young trainee surgeon, I learnt the art, if it can be called an art, of working hard without sleep for prolonged periods. Every doctor has to learn to carry on the next day after an emergency during the previous night. Like everything else you get used to it. I look forward to a real sleep when my day's work is done, but till then I must forget last night and carry on.

It is a common fault of surgeons to remember their successes but conveniently forget their failures. In the heroic pioneering days of surgery when sepsis was common and before the modern armamentarium of blood transfusion, antibiotics, and skilled assistance from the laboratory was as readily available as it is today, it must have been even more difficult to bear the high mortality rates and disappointments which were only too common. Today we are more fortunate, but failure is a condition which all surgeons have to face.

3
An Idea

I was asleep in our house in Limuru one night back in the 1950s when the telephone rang and I was called back to Nairobi to see a Mexican multi-millionaire who had been scragged by a leopard somewhere up-country. A doctor in Nairobi told me the story and produced the wet plates of X-rays of his left knee. There was no fracture but considerable soft tissue injury as I was to discover when I inspected this wound. My patient was lying on a couch in a house in Muthaiga. I was ushered in and informed that this accident had occurred earlier in the same day and he had been flown down to Nairobi by plane. He told me that a leopard had run across a glade and that he had taken a quick shot but had only wounded it. The leopard had turned and come straight for him, knocked him down and started mauling him. The hunter had finally despatched the leopard but this had been difficult because the animal was on top of his client and clearly the hunter was hampered and in danger of shooting the man rather than the animal. A temporary dressing had been put on my patient and somehow they managed to carry him back to the camp. When I looked at the wound, I could see that the knee joint was opened and that he would require an operation. I gave him an injection of penicillin and went out to arrange his admission to hospital. I put him into the old Maia Carberry nursing home, woke up the staff and got them to prepare the theatre.

After a long wait we finally managed to get everything organized and the patient anaesthetized. It appeared as if the wound had been caused by the claws rather than the teeth. Wounds caused by cats are notorious for infection, so I cut away the edges of the wound and any obviously contaminated areas and sewed up the capsule of the joint with some trepidation, and closed the rest of the wound with a series of nylon sutures. I put the whole leg in a plaster cast to immobilize it and help relieve the pain. I got my patient back into his room and left to catch up with some sleep.

In the morning when I called to see how my patient was getting on, I ran into a barrage of his 'hangers-on'. There were his private doctor, his physiotherapist, his secretary, his brother and the son of the President of Mexico among others. I was bombarded with questions. When could he leave hospital? Was he going to lose his leg? Finally, I got in to see the patient. His physical condition seemed satisfactory, his pulse and temperature were normal and the plaster reasonably comfortable. There then ensued the following remarkable conversation.

'Mr Wood,' he said, 'I would like all my food sent up from a restaurant in Nairobi.'

'I am sure that is not necessary,' I replied, 'as the food is very good here, but I will talk to the matron and see what she says.'

'Another matter, Mr Wood. You have not arranged for a private bathroom for me.'

'Mr X, there are no private bathrooms in this hospital. I am sorry, but really you can hardly need a bath as your leg is in plaster.'

His reply to this somewhat truculent remark of mine was a classic.

'Build one,' he said. 'I have the money.'

I realized then that I was in for trouble, and the sooner this gentleman left for Mexico the easier my life would become. I remained at his beck and call for a few days while arrangements were made to transport him back to his home. I managed to keep my temper, but with difficulty. Eventually I was told by one of his minions that he had ordered a private DC6 from Amsterdam with a double KLM crew and that he would be leaving the following day. I secretly breathed a sigh of relief. This was shortlived, however, as I was summoned to his presence again and told that he insisted on me going too and handing him over to his surgeon in Mexico. I remonstrated that this was hardly necessary and that I was very busy. Nothing made any dent on Mr X's expressed wishes. In the end I agreed to go, provided he would pay a large sum to the hospital that we were building in Nairobi. To soften the blow, I told him I would not charge any fees provided my expenses were paid. A cheque-book was produced and he wrote it out but put down only half the figure which we had discussed.

'I will give you the other half in Mexico before you leave.' That was the bargain.

I then had a frantic time rearranging my own commitments, packing and getting ready to go. Susan took me down to the aircraft. We were allowed on to the tarmac in order to deal with the ambulance and my patient. He was lifted aboard, I said goodbye to Susan, who looked somewhat astonished by the whole affair, and shortly we were in the air bound for Paris. I looked around to see who were my companions. There were six of us in this enormous machine; the other members of his staff had been left behind to clear up his house and to follow on later.

I slept most of the way to Paris. My patient's leg still seemed to be behaving well. I gave him his injections and kept him well sedated. It appeared, when we arrived in Paris, that Mr X had taken several floors of the Bristol Hotel. I was allocated a suite which was so large that I almost got lost in it. I scattered my few clothes and private possessions through a maze of cupboards and drawers and went off to find my patient. He was in very affable form and said to me:

'We shall be here a few days while arrangements are made to fly to New York, and I want you to enjoy yourself. My staff will look after you, just tell them what you want to do.'

Rather taken aback at this generous offer, I said, 'That is very kind of you. When would you like to see me again?'

'Come in morning and evening,' he said, 'to see how I am.' I was dismissed.

There ensued three days of riotous living. I was taken to Fontainebleau, to Versailles, to smart restaurants, theatres and night-clubs in rapid succession. Each day I went twice to see my patient. Yes, his plaster was comfortable. No, he had not slept well, could I please change his sleeping pills. My medical job was not arduous.

Once while attending to my patient a knock came on the door and in walked two very smart hotel servants carrying large cardboard boxes.

'Put them down over there in the corner,' said Mr X. They were duly stacked in the corner. Three journeys were necessary before all the boxes had arrived. My curiosity got the better of me.

'What is in all those boxes, Mr X?' I asked in a somewhat abrupt way.

'Oh,' he said, 'I always buy my shirts in Paris.' Before we parted company in Mexico I became quite used to the ways of the very rich. It was to be part of my education.

Another enormous aircraft had been chartered to take us to New York. We left in great style, with what appeared to be the whole hotel staff to see us off. Mr X had arranged a press conference at the airport in New York, although he hadn't seen fit to tell me about this. While transferring into one of his private aircraft at Kennedy Airport, I found myself surrounded by fifty reporters with note-books.

'What happened to Mr X? Did he shoot the leopard? Tell us all the details about his injuries.'

This went on for half an hour or so till I was able finally to escape to Mr X's plane, which I found was lined with leopard skins. I thought this rather ironic but at least the leopards had got their own back. We took off on the long non-stop flight to Mexico City. I found myself in the rear of the aircraft behind Mr X's private cabin being invited to play poker by his staff. We sat in our shirt-sleeves surrounded by this amazing décor, playing cards and whiling away the time. It was an extraordinary situation, but little did I know what was in store for me.

At Mexico City there was a tremendous reception including a band, searchlights and a welcoming committee. It was late in the evening. The hero was duly placed in an ambulance, having held court for half an hour, and was whisked off to his home. Arrangements had been made for me at a neighbouring hotel and I arrived there to find the usual luxury. I had a nasty feeling that perhaps I was getting used to this treatment and that my life in East

Africa would seem very humdrum in comparison.

In the morning a consultation was held with his surgeon and I handed over my patient to his care with my notes and the X-rays. Mr X was in excellent spirits and told me he had arranged for me to have a few days' holiday before leaving for home. I was taken out of his house and there stood a magnificent open red Cadillac with a chauffeur, the President's ADC, a valet and a secretary. I remonstrated with Mr X's secretary and finally managed to dispense with a certain amount of the impedimenta! It was an amazing few days, somewhat akin to a story from *The Arabian Nights*. A repetition of what I did during these days would become irksome and boring. Suffice it to say that I was flown round Mexico in a private P.46, I went deep-sea fishing from the President's yacht and caught several sail-fish and a 240lb. black marlin. I visited his ranch, I went to a bull-fight, and at last was allowed to intimate that it was time I went home.

My last visit to Mr X was one which remains firmly in my memory. Naturally, I thanked him profusely for his great generosity and after wishing him a rapid recovery, I broached the subject of the other half of his donation to the hospital in Nairobi. I was determined to extract this before leaving.

'Well,' said Mr X, 'business has not been very good and my staff tell me that I have very little money.'

I was so astonished by this remark that before I had time to think I heard myself saying, 'Mr X, your secretary has just told me you ordered a private Comet' (the jet airliner that was causing such a stir at the time). 'Surely you would like to keep your promise to me,' I said, standing over him at the bedside. His response was to roar with laughter.

'Well,' he said, 'I must obviously sack my secretary, but here is the cheque. I just wanted to test you out.' Having been duly tested, I left with a ticket on which this kind gentleman said I could go anywhere in the world on my way home. I visited California, took in the Mayo Clinic at Rochester, Minnesota and finally arrived back in Nairobi. It was high time I tackled the real problems of life in Africa again.

One day after my return from abroad I was telephoned by a businessman in Nairobi who asked me to go up and see a desperately ill man in Hargesia, in what was then British Somaliland. It was a trip of fifteen hundred miles each way. I was asked to bring a physician with me, and Dr Charters, a specialist physician, agreed to come. We hired a Miles Magister, collected our medical kit and instruments, and set off. I was not flying myself so I had time to ponder on the medical use of aeroplanes and also have a close look at the countryside. We had decided to fly to Mogadishu, the capital of Italian Somaliland, in order to be able to refuel before going off to Hargesia. No one who flies over Africa can be anything but astonished at the hundreds of miles which pass below one in which there appears to be no human habitation. Much of this land is dry waterless bush but there are still enormous areas awaiting development and food production for the hungry world. One of the first major landmarks was the Tana River which we came to at Garissa, where we could pinpoint our exact position. There were no radio beacons in those days. This river is now being used for hydro-electric power and for irrigation projects and will play an ever-increasing part in the agricultural life of Kenya. Then on over the desert until we hit the Juba River and finally the coast south of Mogadishu, and followed this up till we saw the white buildings of the capital city of Somaliland. The Indian Ocean is always a joy to see, particularly after hours of travel over the desert. It gave me the feeling that travellers must get when they sight the oasis after a long trek over the sand. It so happened that day that there was a riot going on in Mogadishu. We couldn't discover what it was about but the end result was that we couldn't get Shell to refuel us. Everyone was staying indoors and from time to time a rifle was let off and occasionally we heard the staccato sound of a machine-gun. We decided to stay the night in town and see if we could get fuel in the morning. Finally we persuaded a taxi to take us to a hotel. The roads were full of shouting people, but we got through unscathed and never really discovered what all the fuss was about. We were up early in the morning, managed to extricate the Shell attendants, and shortly afterwards took to the sky, somewhat relieved that we were on our way again. Hargesia is not an easy place to find without navigational aids and radio, and the atmosphere was full of sand so there was very little forward visibility. Our navigator, however, did an extremely good job and brought us in without any trouble. It had been a monotonous flight but it all helped me to frame in my mind the medical problems of these isolated places. We were met by the

Army doctor who had been looking after our patient and from him we got the story. Some three weeks before this man had been taken ill in Berbera on the coast where he was the managing director of a large business. He had gone to bed and been seen by a doctor there who had prescribed for him. The diagnosis was apparently never certain but he had had severe abdominal pain and vomiting. As he did not get better, he was transferred by ambulance up the long road to Hargesia. By the time he arrived he was unconscious and had remained so now for over a week. Dr Charters and I examined him and found that he had a mass on the right side of his abdomen and a large tender liver. He also had a high swinging temperature, a high white blood cell count and clearly there was an acute infective process going on. We managed to get him X-rayed, which showed some distended loops of intestine and the large liver, but nothing else of great significance. We put the various pieces of the jig-saw together and came to the conclusion that he had had an attack of appendicitis which had gone on to abscess formation, portal pyaemia and abscesses in the liver. It looked as if we were up against an insuperable problem, as indeed it turned out to be. He had been given a blood transfusion, penicillin and all the correct treatment but it was really too late. I took him to the theatre and put a large needle into his liver to confirm the diagnosis. I drew out a quantity of evil-smelling pus. This clinched the diagnosis and we felt certain that he could not survive, as there were multiple abscesses and his liver was virtually destroyed. Sadly he died shortly afterwards, and never recovered consciousness. It taught me another lesson that speed in these cases is essential. So often one is called in when really it is too late and one can only support one's colleague while the patient dies. It is true that the responsibility is shared in this way and one can comfort the doctor in telling him that he could not have done anything more in the circumstances. This is cold comfort and often I have wished to have been called earlier to similar cases. After a night under canvas we returned over the same route, disappointed but perhaps wiser. If cost is considered in these cases, it is, of course, an expensive business. On this occasion it was of no great importance as the expenses involved were paid by the company, who could well afford it. Two specialists and two aircrew had been involved, three thousand miles travelled and very little accomplished. However, where human life is at stake an effort has to be made and even if it ends in failure, as on this occasion, perhaps something is notched up on the final score and humanity is redeemed to some small degree.

Africa is a very large continent and for the time being specialist skills are at a premium. Good radio communication, in the absence of telephones, can prevent fruitless journeys, especially when the doctor on the spot can talk to a colleague hundreds of miles away and give him the latest condition of a sick patient. It is also possible then to go with the knowledge of what equipment is required and whether certain drugs or blood for transfusion are needed. Cables are often useless and tend to arrive after the man who has sent the cable in the first place. Crossing national boundaries has, sadly, become more difficult in recent years and the formalities involved are often time-consuming and wasteful when lives are at stake and time is of the essence.

It was this flight which I had undertaken as a private person which made me think about the possible advantages of starting a service to visit these remote places in the bush. The idea of using the aeroplane for extending medical services appealed to me and it seemed then that East Africa was tailor-made for this type of approach. It would need some clear thinking if a practical plan was to be formulated, but the germ of an idea had been planted in my mind and there it remained as a chimera or utopian dream to be played with in my imagination over the coming years. It was later to be watered and fed by my own experience and that of my friends, but at the moment the problems of insufficient money and time were enough to keep the idea well in the background and beyond the bounds of possibility.

It was about now that we decided we wanted to take up farming in a bigger way. We had become so intrigued with the life, but the farm wasn't big enough to make any money and school fees started to become a major item in our budget, so we felt we should try and supplement my income and build up an asset for the future.

We had been introduced to life on Kilimanjaro by Robin Johnston, who was a close friend of Archie McIndoe. He had enthused us with the pioneering life and when the opportunity presented itself we bought the next-door farm to his and sold the farm at Limuru. Our association with Archie McIndoe turned into a very real and important friendship. He would arrive out on his farm on Kilimanjaro every year to join Robin in bringing in the wheat harvest. He would stay with us in Nairobi on his way and often we would end up on the farm together to enjoy the magnificent air and scenery and the unique experience of turning the African bush into fruitful wheatland. These were wonderful days which were gilded by Archie's enthusiasm and sense of humour. Great surgeon that he was he could not come to Africa without seeing what needed to be done surgically. Of an evening around the log fire with our beers in our hands and our shoes off, we would talk about this. One year Archie brought with him a young American surgeon, Tom Rees, who caught the magic of Africa and its compelling problems. The three of us finally laid the plans which materialized into a Foundation, and to this day Tom pays us a yearly visit and gives of his skills to Africa and keeps a guiding hand on the committee in America.

We went back to live in Nairobi during the week-time but managed to get to the new farm at the weekends. And so started a new chapter which was to lead to twenty years of adventurous living in what must be one of the most beautiful places on this earth.

4
The Farm

I found farming the perfect antidote to my medical job, and the idea of carving out a piece of Africa and watching things grow had always been an ambition of mine. As it turned out, I had this idea but Susan did all the work and over the years made a solid success of it. Again the aeroplane played an important part in our lives and without it I would never have contemplated the move. It enabled me to get to the farm at the weekends and the change of scene and activity helped me keep a sense of proportion. For the children it was a wonderful find. What more could one ask for than a wonderful climate, plenty of room to move around, fishing, shooting, and the safari life at close hand? The only disadvantage of being brought up in these circumstances is that you suffer from claustrophobia anywhere else. The wide open spaces have such a compelling enchantment, and as Susan made a lovely home for us all we tried always to get back there whether we were at work, travelling the world, or at school.

Some people have the knack of nest building – Susan had this art to a high degree. Making a home cosy, being an imaginative cook, designing a new garden, are all part of her nature so the children always flocked home as birds to a nest. It was a wonderful upbringing and now that they have flown the nest to make their own lives, part of their hearts, a very deep part, will always return to Ol Molog to relive its joys, its beauty and its memories. I know in my own heart that it will haunt them all their lives as something almost too good to be true, something to be savoured for all time. I have made many rash decisions in my life but going to Ol Molog is one I shall never regret and nor, I believe, will the family.

I used to feel the magnetic pull of my home as I dealt with the last patient in Nairobi and got into the aeroplane and headed south. Often it was late and I had a battle against the fall of darkness. The airstrip was on Robin's farm, only three-quarters of a mile from our house. The discipline of flying is such that despite the hurry I made myself do the checks on the aircraft, as I instinctively knew that this was an insurance against the human error which can so easily creep in. To run out of fuel in an aircraft is something that no one will forgive you for, including yourself. Familiarity breeds contempt and this is the ever-present danger in flying.

The Twin Comanche was looking sleek and purposeful as I walked round her familiarizing myself with her shape and recalling the various checks which I was meant to do. I had put in a flight plan and disciplined myself to take this flight without any hurry so that I should not make any stupid mistakes, as I was tired after the week's work. I checked the oil, the tyres, those hinges in the ailerons which are so vital, and the elevators, and I ran my hand along the leading edges and the propeller, almost like stroking a favourite dog. When I had satisfied myself about the outside of the aircraft, I jumped into the cockpit and sat there for a time admiring the compact design of the instrument panel. I did up my seat belt, closed and locked the door and slowly let my eyes accustom themselves to the position of the dials and switches. I turned on the master switch and the radios and asked for start-up clearance from the control tower. This was granted. On went the magneto switches, mixtures rich, propeller in fine pitch, fuel on to both tanks. Then fuel pumps on to prime the engine and press the starter – there was immediate response and my eyes watched the oil-pressure gauge – the pressure came up quickly. Now for the starboard engine – the same drill and again instant response. I throttled both engines back to idle and called the tower again. I was cleared to taxi. I started to move forward, checked on the brakes and then slowly moved off along the taxi way. There was very little wind but what there was came from the east. The 07 runway was in use and several aircraft came in as I proceeded slowly to the threshold. Right – do your run up and cockpit drill. Can I remember it? It comes back almost automatically. Revs up to 1800 on both engines, check the magnetos, pull the prop levers back and then forward again not to lose more than 500 revs. Lean the mixture out till the engine starts to run rough and then richen the mixture again. Power checks satisfactory. Check the temperatures – engines are still cold, adjust the trim tabs, magnetos and mixture have been checked. Fuel gauges register full, main tanks on – switch on the electric fuel pumps, 10° of flap on. Check the pressures again, switches all on, safety belts on, doors locked, pull back on the control column, move it to both sides – controls full and free. Take a final look round and call the tower, 'Ready for take-off.' 'Cleared for take-off.' I eased the plane forward, pointed it down the runway and opened the throttles slowly. The glorious surge of power took place which I could feel in my back and neck. Check you are getting full power on the ground – in no time the plane is up to its take-off speed and I eased back the stick – the nose rose and then the wheels unstuck and I was in the air. Keep the nose down to get up to minimum safe single-engine speed, flip up the undercarriage switch, raise the flaps at three hundred feet and she's away. Throttle back a little, adjust the propeller and lean her out as altitude is gained. Swing round to starboard and make for the visual marker. Look out for other aircraft on the circuit. The ritual is almost complete as I level out at 6500 feet and make for the control-zone boundary fifteen nautical miles out. Steer 197° and fly for five minutes on this course. Call Wilson tower on 118·1 and say I am at the control-zone boundary – instructed to go over to 118·5 frequency and call Eastair Centre. I conform and then start to steer 165° and make for Kilimanjaro.

I flew the trip to Ol Molog and back nearly eight hundred times but each time I tried to give it the attention which any cross-country trip deserves. It used to take just over the hour in the Tripacer but in the Twin Comanche I got it down to under forty minutes. It is a wonderful flight and I often noticed when flying guests down to the farm that they too felt the excitement. The first few miles are over the Nairobi National Park and often we saw lions and other game as we gained height and set course for Kilimanjaro. The lions were easily spotted because they were always surrounded by a ring of cars whose occupants were getting a close look at these lazy creatures. On past Kajiado, the administrative centre of the eastern part of Kenya Maasailand. At certain times of the year, and depending on the grazing, the plains here were covered in game and sometimes we were lucky enough to see a rhino or a cheetah. Then came the hills which stretched down towards Amboseli and its famous park. Sand rivers wandered across the landscape and at times carried enormous amounts of water which had run down from the hills after heavy rain. Often I saw herds of elephant at this point onwards, and on the far side of Amboseli, buffalo. This all added to the enchantment as the shadows lengthened and the African dusk fell over this old scene which must have looked the same since the Creation. There is so little interference from man, a Maasai manyatta here and a small road there but essentially the landscape is unchanged. At the moment around 6.15 in the evening the summit of Kilimanjaro would appear. Visitors who had not seen it before often looked for it at too low a level and could scarcely believe its size when their eyes finally focused on it. It rises from the Amboseli plains through forest, moorland and rock to its impressive flat snow-covered top. The clouds evaporate in the evening, casting off their veil to reveal the highest point in Africa. Many are the tales told about this massive mountain so that its very name reminds us of its mysterious quality. 'I will lift up mine eyes unto the hills' – the psalmist understood the healing quality of the hills.

At last I can see Ol Molog on its own shelf lying between the desert below and the forest and snow above – superbly situated like a jewel in a beautiful setting.

Up over the village above the arable land. I start to farm in my mind. What is that tractor doing? Why are the cows grazing in that field? I must talk to Susan about that. Steady – watch what you are doing – you are flying an aeroplane, there is plenty of time for farming later. Below me the tidy fields stretch away, the little extinct volcanoes break the slope, the forest farms, the upper boundary, and then round over the house and in to land between the fields of wheat. The moment I switch off the engine the peace of Ol Molog descends on me, and as I get out of my seat the cool alpine air envelops me. I take a deep breath; I am home. I scarcely have time to take in the magic of the place when

I am whisked off to the house across the farm roads. The wheat looks nearly ripe—when are we going to harvest? What do you expect the yields to be? Avidly I question Susan about the week's work. She is calm and somehow fits into the seasons and the natural order of things. She has that innate ability to put down roots and flourish in the climate of what she creates, calling up her inner reserves for peace, quietude and contentment. Her family feel this instinctively and at once come under her spell.

Engushai was the Maasai name given to the farm and was thought to be the word which describes the parting in the hair. The farm was partially enclosed by a parting in the forest and hence its name. A forest fire raged there in 1912 in the days of German East Africa and burnt out a strip of forest which later became the Ol Molog farms. Certainly when we came to cultivate it there were endless stumps and roots which had to be dragged out, a time-consuming and expensive operation. Ol Molog itself means 'the pimples' in Maasai and describes the secondary volcanoes which were such a distinct feature of the countryside.

One of these little volcanoes was called Loikitoip and from the top of it you could get a panoramic view of the farms and above them the forest and then Kilimanjaro itself. We had two rainy seasons at Ol Molog and we cultivated half the farm in one season and the other half in the other season. The cultivations ran across the farm in strips about thirty yards wide which was the swathe an aircraft could cover with spray in one run. From Loikitoip this pattern gave the farms a zebra-like look, the lighter stripes being the wheat or stubble and the darker stripes the cultivated fallow. This method of farming also helped to break up the fields and prevent wash during heavy rainstorms. This was a problem because the land fell through eight hundred feet over two-and-a-half miles and the water had to go downhill somewhere. We found that harrowing in the stubble after the rain returned some goodness into the soil and helped the texture. It was wonderful dark-red forest loam and its fertility proved to be exceptional.

As we looked out from our vantage point on the volcano with the help of field-glasses, we could pick out the homesteads with their gardens, the flowering cape chestnut trees, the cows in their paddocks and the tractors at work in the fields. It was the place to take visitors because the whole history of development lay before them and each little area of interest could be pointed out and explained. Often we would run down the steep side of the hill as the sun went down and the final pink light left the snow 13,000 feet above us. It was possible, too, to drive up the hill on a steep perilous track provided you had a four-wheel drive and a head for heights.

Each farm had to be as self-sufficient as possible, though we borrowed each other's machinery from time to time. We soon realized the great advantages of bringing up a family on a farm. There were so many things for the children to do and see, and often there were excitements like dealing with elephants in the wheat or spraying the little dioch birds which sometimes came like locusts in their millions to eat the wheat. On the farm we generated our own electricity, piped new sources of water from the forest springs above, and lived off the meat, the vegetables, the fruit and the dairy products. At least once a week someone would drive into Moshi or Arusha to buy groceries, pick up the spare parts and do the farm business. It was a long drive of over sixty miles and at least half the journey was over earth roads which became almost impossible during the rains. Moshi was 3000 feet lower and therefore much hotter, and it was always a great moment in the day when the car started up the farm road and the cool fresh mountain air welcomed the jaded travellers. On getting out of the car you walked on springy green turf and could enjoy again the profusion of flowers and the lovely indigenous forest trees. It was a cool green oasis perched above the dusty arid plains of Amboseli below.

We would often watch the sun go down in the west through the silhouetted tracing of the wild olive trees, and be able to pick out the distant hills like Ol Donyo Lengai as they merged with the lengthening shadows. In Africa this is always a bewitching moment; the wind drops, the temperature drops, the birds fly in to roost and the atmosphere is like black velvet. We would then move into the living-room and start the wood fire and gather round to discuss the day, its joys and its problems. The African staff and their families lived close by in a village which we had built on the farm. The head man, Joshua, would often come in and report on the work and discuss with Susan their plans for the following day. These men had a great feel for the place and there was no patronizing attitude towards them. They were part of the team and I believe honestly enjoyed the life there as much as we did. Often Susan would be over in the village dosing one of the children, and they would all flock round her, as she was a great favourite, dealing with them as she would with her own children. They sensed that she was part of the Africa they knew, kindly, quiet and yet with an indefinable authority.

When I look back at our time there, I become conscious that it was the atmosphere which made this place unique for us. This atmosphere was made by a mixture of many ingredients which included the companionship of good friends, the tackling of a new enterprise, the beautiful scenery around Kilimanjaro, and the moulding of a new way of life which was immensely worthwhile and stimulating. All these elements together formed a special blend of experience, something which was felt by our visitors as much as by ourselves.

The bracing air made us all feel so well, although I suspect that the high altitude gave rise to bouts of what we called 'high-altitude neurosis' which ran through the community from time to time and were fortunately soon forgotten. It made us make mountains out of molehills, a kind of hysteria charged with heat and very little light. For some people Ol Molog might seem to be out in the backwoods and very remote, as it was a long way from the nearest town and at the end of the line of communications. There was a remarkable telephone system in which we all shared the same party line. Nothing was secret or confidential and the whole neighbourhood knew everybody else's business. It was also suspected that certain people took great delight in listening in to other people's conversation – talk about the 'bush telegraph'! The situation became hilarious but as long as one remembered not to discuss anything of real importance on the telephone no one suffered. There were all sorts of variations on the theme, as it was intriguing to say something outrageous on the phone and see how long it took to come back to roost. You then knew who had been listening in. We each had separate rings : for instance, ours was two longs and a short, and you then knew who was being called.

Tapping of telephones, I am told, is done all over the world and not only by the CIA, but in our case it was unnecessary as every call was like addressing a public meeting anyhow.

The West Kilimanjaro Club, twenty miles down the road, was another splendid institution. I used to refer to it as 'Dodge City

1870', as somehow I always expected the sheriff to walk in and there to be fisticuffs at the bar and someone shooting out the light. Saturday nights were the time when a fair proportion of us farmers would resort to the Club to exchange stories, compare each other's harvests and spread rumours of unbelievable proportions. There was a great sense of camaraderie and everything else was usually taken in good part and 'mobbing up' was the order of the day. If ever I heard someone say, 'Do you know what I heard at the Club last Saturday?', I divided the ensuing piece of news by ten in order to allow for the inevitable exaggeration.

It was a great place for blowing off steam, seeing other members of the community and having a game of darts. People used to come out from Moshi and Arusha to join in the innocent fun and its popularity proved it was a worthwhile enterprise. It was quite a distance from Ol Molog, which meant that those farthest along the line had quite a safari to make, and in the rain they could end up in a long walk home after the car had slid into the ditch.

The use of aeroplanes reduced the isolation and most of us at Ol Molog used them as they were cheaper than cars to run and much quicker. Farm spares during harvest were fetched rapidly and essential visits to Nairobi on business were easily accomplished. The airstrip at our end of Ol Molog was constructed in the early days and proved to be excellent, though some of our passengers used to suggest, when they saw how narrow the strip was, that we might have been a little more generous with its width and less greedy about growing wheat so close to the edges.

Our family life at Engushai was never dull as there were so many comings and goings. Mark and Hugo went to a preparatory school at Gilgil in Kenya and then on to public schools in England. It was a wrench for them to be packed off thousands of miles away and they used to return with pale faces and stories of their scholastic endeavours which they never found easy, but finally they scraped through their exams and were able to put them behind them and launch out on their careers. Mark collected butterflies, which took him running round the countryside and forest, while Hugo became interested in birds, which were one of the many bonuses of life on Kilimanjaro. There were some four hundred species varying from the large predator eagles and buzzards down to the tiny sun birds, and though East Africa is perhaps best known for its wild game, it is also a unique place for the bird watchers.

The girls, Janet and Katrina, went through the well-known riding stage when everything else is cast aside and horses become the passion of the moment. It was an ideal place for this occupation and the horizons were limitless. During the holidays we would sometimes take off for the low country with a picnic breakfast to shoot game birds. The sand grouse would come in to drink at the furrow which brought down water from the slopes of Mount Meru out into the dry country where the game and Maasai cattle abounded. After getting our barrels red hot we would find a special place in one of the sand rivers and build a roaring fire on which we brewed hot water for tea, and made a delicious mixture of scrambled eggs and sausages while reclining in the shade of a tree. After this interlude we would set forth again after yellow-neck francoline, guinea-fowl, duck and geese. We seldom had to buy meat as the birds and an occasional buck on the farm kept the larder full. It was good exercise trying to keep up with the guinea-fowl as the sun rose and with it the temperature. The geese very often outwitted us and seemed to know instinctively how to keep out of range of our shotguns. Occasionally we were fortunate but we had to be well hidden to stand a chance with these wily birds. It was always a great delight to be down in the savannah country and we would come across eland, giraffe, oryx, lesser kudu, and sometimes even lions were around. We would wend our way back up the mountain, tired and hot, and after lunch sleep would often overtake us as a result of the fresh air, exercise and food. These days are often recalled as memory of them lingers on.

Like other families we would occasionally have violent arguments, usually about totally unimportant issues. The game Monopoly brought out the worst in us all and we each accused each other of cheating, while our determination to build yet another hotel took over from our sense of humour and our tempers frayed. Sue and I would then suggest doing something different to help cool off the heat and it would usually end with equanimity being restored. Music, too, played a valuable part in our leisure hours as we all appreciated it, though we were very poor performers. The exquisite recordings which are available today, the records and tapes, perhaps discourage any attempt to compete and we have become a society of listeners, and viewers of television.

Holidays and term-time flew by and finally even university struggles were over. Mark studied medicine, Janet social anthropology, Hugo agriculture and Katrina philosophy and French. When we had passed through this expensive performance Sue and I mistakenly thought that we were out of the wood. We were soon to be confounded. While launching our brood on their chosen careers we were overtaken by weddings, homes, travel, equipment and motor cars, which seemed to be required in an unending stream. It was an investment which we never regretted and perhaps supporting a family and getting them on the first rung of the ladder is the most fulfilling way of buying one's immortality. They have all repaid us many times over by their successes and by their companionship for their ageing parents.

Our enterprise at Ol Molog flourished largely due to Sue's constant care of it and then to Robin and Hugo's expert management. Robin, our son-in-law, was an expert with machinery and had learnt to farm because it was in his blood. He had been born and bred on a farm in Tanzania and he had watched his father at work and managed other farms while building up his experience. He was always popular with the labour because he could jockey them along and make them laugh, but, above all, he could do all the jobs himself and his example was the most convincing factor in his make-up. Janet, our daughter, had a bright academic mind and a great love for the African wild. School and university in England had only served to convince her that she wanted to spend her life where she had been brought up. This is a common finding among European children brought up in East Africa and many of them find it very difficult to settle in the more crowded industrial countries. Janet became very expert with the business side of the farm and the accounts and made a great contribution in this way to the family enterprise.

Hugo, our younger son, had struggled through a degree in agriculture at Wye and then came back to manage the next-door farm. At once he found his rightful place and blossomed quickly into a competent practical farmer. He was debonair, popular, hard-working and driven mad by any bureaucracy. His political views at one time were described as slightly to the right of

Genghis Khan! With this team behind her Susan had all the ingredients of success. She was the one who did many of the less glamorous jobs on the farm but she was a counsellor and friend to so many and she formed the matrix which stuck the whole enterprise together. At one moment she would be treating a child with pneumonia – at the next she would be at a meeting with the accountants or telephoning for spare parts or gardening or looking after visitors. It was twelve hours on the go most days for her, but she was her own boss and she thrived on the variety of her tasks and responsibilities.

In most ways it was an ideal life, and when the farming jobs were done there were so many wonderful places to visit. We used to enjoy the bird-shooting, the trout-fishing on the mountain and visits to the game parks or to the coast. The outdoor life was incomparable and spoilt us for life almost anywhere else. The charm of East African life was immortalized by Karen Blixen nearly fifty years ago in her book, *Out of Africa*[1], which describes the atmosphere so beautifully and brings feelings of nostalgia to all East Africans.

We were able to buy the next-door farm and finally an eight-thousand-acre ranch some twenty miles away. This gave the boys enough room to work on their own particular interests, without treading on each other's toes. I loved the lower farm as a contrast to the Ol Molog farms. It was warmer down there and had its own particular African magic. At certain times of year it had over two thousand head of game on it, apart from our eight hundred head of beef cattle. We had a herd of some seventy oryx which were an especial delight and there were always giraffe and the other plains game and often elephant, buffalo, rhino, lion and leopard. Big game and farming are incompatible particularly if there is arable land, as a herd of elephant can lay waste a field of wheat in a very short time. As a result of man's expansion in farming, the areas where game can roam freely are being encroached on and this inevitably leads to a decrease in the total game population. When in the mood over the weekend, I would drive down to the lower farm and wander around on the ranch enjoying my own game park and absorbing the pleasures of farming in Africa and then return in the cool of the evening up the

[1] *Out of Africa*, Karen Blixen, Putnams, 1937.

road to Ol Molog. I was badly addicted to Africa, a serious afflic-
tion for which there is no known cure. It is a chronic complaint
which once it has struck never leaves you alone. It is felt most
strongly when you are away in one of the industrialized countries. The claustrophobia begins to attack you; you pine for the
warm sun, the smell of thorn trees in blossom, the clarity of the
air and the noises of the African night. This intangible yet powerful sensation makes you yearn to return and bury yourself once
more in its compelling embrace. It is a life-long love story which
has no end. I have seen many people leave Africa for one reason
or another but directly they have taken the fatal step the malady
takes hold of them and never lets them go. When I am out of
Africa I sometimes try to diagnose the condition but I never get
close to the real truth. Is it the climate? Is it living on the
equator? Is it the intoxication of the senses, the sight, the taste,
the smell? It is none of these things; it is more subtle, more
numbing, more all-pervasive and more deadly. Perhaps it is similar
to the condition to which the lotus eaters succumbed. Could they
describe what they felt? It is best to give in to it and simply
return again to Africa, which alone can assuage the pangs. Home
sickness can only be cured by returning home.

Archie McIndoe and Tom Rees felt just the same as we did
about Africa in general and Ol Molog in particular. Perhaps it
was not surprising then that this atmosphere helped us to think
of medical development at the same time. There was so much
to do but we needed a vehicle to carry forward our ideas, and
so when we returned to our places of work Tom gathered some
of his friends together in New York and set up a legal entity called
the African Research Foundation and Archie started a charitable
organization in London with the same name and working out of
the Royal College of Surgeons. I busied myself with setting up
a committee in Nairobi of interested people and Lord Twining
kindly took on the chairmanship, and in time we registered it
again as the African Research Foundation. At this moment in time
we might, if we had given it thought, have been somewhat
daunted at the task we had undertaken. We had an idea, no
money, and a whole continent to work in; not really a good
combination to start with, but it certainly allowed plenty of
scope.

The concept that Archie, Tom and I envisaged in the early days has, of course, been modified in the light of our experience and the Foundation we started has taken on many tasks along the road.

Communications were an early focal point and from these we went on to creating departments in health education, mobile medicine on the ground, surgery, training, printing, publications and research. Around these departments a strong administrative and accounts section grew to cope with the expanding staff, accounting to donors and all the many jobs which needed to be done to keep the Foundation on the straight and narrow path. An information office, a projects officer and finally an administrator of our consultancy services were added and the organization on the ground which had started with one man had, by 1977, grown to a staff of sixty people.

While all these plans were being discussed and gradually implemented, I continued to explore on my own the possibilities of using aircraft in the service of rural people and I made many sorties into the bush and two right across Africa to the West Coast and back. Slowly I learnt some of the intuitive skills of the bush pilot – the flying by one's shirt-tails, as it is called.

5
In the Air

The idea of running a medical service by air and what has come to be known as the Flying Doctor Service grew slowly. Such a service had been pioneered and run most successfully in Australia and there was nothing original in the idea – it was simply the same concept of using the aeroplane and the radio as a tool in the planning of medical services to the remote areas. The Rev. Flynn, the founder of the Royal Australian Flying Doctor Service, had used the phrase, 'throwing a mantle of safety over the continent'. Somehow this seemed to be a very apt expression and in the minds of the public this concept is readily understood. In our case, the Flying Doctor Service helped to transport not only patients and medical and nursing staff, but also radio engineers, training staff and anyone in the Foundation who was working in the field or supervising our growing number of projects.

The first gift of an aeroplane which the Foundation received was a Piper Aztec from Arthur Godfrey in the USA. It was immediately useful and a great improvement on my own private aeroplane, as it could carry more people and equipment and cover the ground much faster.

I then had to face the problem of building airfields on which our aircraft could land, and at suitable places close to the medical facility we were trying to help. This task proved easier than anticipated and was largely due to the manual work which the local African people contributed freely to this enterprise. Once the local authorities understood that we wanted an airfield to bring in doctors and nurses to treat them there was usually no trouble, and with the guidance of a pilot a suitable stretch of land was selected and then cleared. The strip had to face into the prevailing wind, be at least six hundred yards long, and have unobstructed approaches. Usually the surface was grass, though in the drier areas sand or murram were the order of the day.

On one occasion, nine thousand men working for a day produced a strip one thousand yards long on which I landed the same evening to evacuate a seriously injured patient. I have to admit I have landed on better strips – this one went up and down like a scenic railway and on landing I was thrown into the air again by two mounds which were not visible except from the ground. However, the mission was accomplished without incident and the making of airstrips has been one of the real contributions which the local people have made and continue to make.

It is less easy to get these strips maintained and the grass cut. The aeroplane is no longer a novelty; they had been seen to land safely many times, so why bother to cut the grass? Over the years, we have gradually had the strips lengthened and by constant appeals and threats most of them are maintained to a safe standard.

Wild animals or the domestic cow or goat appearing out of the bushes just as the pilot is fully committed to land can be a hazard. Holes are dug by wild pigs or ant bears, so we like to have the strips inspected before an aircraft lands – another good use for the radio network. The condition of the strip can be radioed to the pilot before he lands or even before he starts on his journey. Occasionally in our system of over one hundred strips, one of them may get flooded or a tree falls across it and news about this is, of course, vital to the safety of the aircraft.

All East African pilots have tales to tell of the near-misses they have had with wild animals and other disasters. One incident stands out in my mind involving a rhino which I spotted on the strip on which I was going to land. After a few low passes to try and persuade this large animal to move off, I managed to get him to the far end of the strip. I then landed short and kept a weather eye on the old fellow, who promptly trotted towards my plane to investigate this rude intrusion. I felt rather stupid and undecided what to do. Fortunately I had not shut off the engine so I opened the throttle, which made a great din. This stopped the rhino in his tracks, but as I closed the throttle again he started to advance once more. By this time there was not enough room to take off over the rhino so I decided that attack was the best form of defence. I taxied towards him and wished I had had a horn to blow, but they don't fit these to aircraft. My shouting 'Go away, you big brute' was clearly not going to be heard above the engine noise, so I abandoned this ploy and put my faith in total confrontation. It worked; the rhino turned tail and trotted off down the strip in high dudgeon, and I turned round and was glad to see the car which had come out to pick me up approaching through a cloud of dust. I left my aircraft at the end of the strip and hoped the rhino would not investigate any closer. I then turned to more serious matters and soon had forgotten the incident as I listened to the medical problems which were the cause of my visit.

For a long time there had been thoughts about trying to construct an airstrip to serve Ortum Hospital in the Marech pass in North-West Kenya. It was difficult terrain with mountains rising steeply out of the valley on either side. The valley was narrow, stony and uneven. Father Staples of the Mission there who had started the school and hospital, was convinced it could be done: I was less sure. As it turned out he was right and I was wrong.

I flew up to Kitale and drove down the road from Kapenguria which never runs straight for more than fifty yards; twisting and turning it eventually comes out at Sigor in the Kerio Valley at a much lower altitude. The scenery is exciting as on the right are the Cherangani mountains running up to 11,000 feet through green forest, and on the left are rocky mountains which are not so high but steep and barren. Occasionally there is a stream to cross as the road winds downhill and finally opens on to the valley floor, which runs north and south and is a parallel off-shoot of the Great Rift Valley. Down the Kerio River comes the rain-water from the Cheranganis and surrounding highlands, and flash floods in this river can suddenly cause great difficulties for the hospital at Lokori farther downstream by making the crossing impossible and cutting them off for days from their sources of supply to the south. Finally the Kerio opens into the west side of Lake Turkana, the Jade Sea, which is the great feature of the northern deserts of Kenya.

Father Staples and I had a good look round the valley and the more I saw of it the less I liked it. The wind in the Marech Pass gets up around ten o'clock in the morning and blows up the pass strongly all day, fading away as the sun goes down. After much discussion, I said to Father Staples:

'I bet you cannot make an airstrip here six hundred yards long by November 12th.' I mentioned this date because I had a German television team coming to Nairobi and I wanted to have some shots taken of a bush airstrip under construction.

'All right,' said Father Staples. 'If I get the strip made will you bring an aeroplane in?'

I was now on the spot. Father Staples teased me by saying that the Flying Doctor pilots were a timid lot and would only land on major fields. He had said this deliberately to persuade me to accept the challenge. I felt fairly confident that he could not make the strip and certainly within the time, as November 12th was only a few weeks ahead. So I accepted the challenge on one condition, that I could look at the strip on the ground again to see it was safe before landing. I went back to Nairobi and really forgot about it as other matters pressed in on me and kept me fully occupied.

To my surprise I got a message after a few weeks to say the airstrip was ready and when was I going to bring the aeroplane? I went up again to Ortum and found they had done a fantastic job. Father Staples had secured the help of the African District Commissioner and had got the loan of a bulldozer and grader. This had made all the difference. I had thought that the work would have to be done by hand. I had underestimated Father Staples's influence, ingenuity and determination. There had been great boulders at the eastern end of the strip and as I walked down the strip to test the surface I was amazed to see that these boulders, weighing many tons, had disappeared. They had built fires on them with sticks and logs and when they got very hot, had struck them with hammers and split off pieces which they had carried away. This had been a formidable undertaking. I had not known this technique and would not have believed it possible unless I had seen it with my own eyes. I paced out the strip, six hundred and fifty yards in all; it ran uphill for most of its length and then finally flattened out for a hundred yards or so before coming to some high trees and an impossible ditch just before the hospital grounds. The strip was perfectly placed for the use of the hospital as it was so close and within two or three minutes' walking distance. I made another tour of the strip. The grader was still at work. We got some ridges and humps taken out and a promise that the windsock would be ready and finally arranged the day for the official opening of the strip, which was to be done by our friend the District Commissioner. Father Staples now had me cornered and he clearly enjoyed the situation. My main problem was the landing, because I reckoned I could only land uphill and unfortunately this would mean landing with the wind. The trees at the far end and the considerable slope of the runway made it unwise, in my judgement, to attempt to come in the other way. Another factor involved the impossibility of overshooting once committed to the landing in the valley floor. It was also impossible to turn the aircraft as the valley was so narrow at the level of its floor.

The day came for the attempt. A radio had been installed at Ortum so we were able to ascertain that we had a fine day for the opening ceremony. In the early afternoon I arrived overhead in the valley with two members of the television team aboard, duly provided with their cameras and sound equipment. Flying at a considerable height above Ortum, I noticed at once that the windsock was completely horizontal, indicating a wind of thirty m.p.h. up the valley in the only direction I could land. Lining the strip were hundreds and hundreds of the local tribesmen and I could see the Sisters in white looking up at the aircraft. Well, here we go, I thought, as I worked out my tactics. I had to fly down the valley losing height and then turn through 180° while there was still room to do so and creep up the valley and drop the aircraft on the very first few feet of the runway if I was to have a chance of stopping before running into the trees at the far end. As I did my turn and approached the threshold of the strip I realized I was going much too fast for comfort with the wind giving me an extra thirty m.p.h. With this feeling came the knowledge that I was now committed and had to put the aeroplane down. There was no viable alternative. I touched down going over 80 m.p.h. and the far end of the strip came into view almost at once. The uphill run had slowed me down a lot and

I had been able to use the brakes, though not strongly, as I was worried about skidding in the soft sand which had been left by the grader. The trees became alarmingly close – I kicked the rudder hard to the left and did a sort of christi and then came to a standstill. The crowds rushed to the aeroplane directly it was standing still. I felt sure that someone would be decapitated by the propeller. The cameraman went on filming the eager black faces pressed against the windows. Having turned off all the switches, we struggled out against an avalanche of human bodies which threatened to crush us back against the fuselage. Father Staples and the Sisters came to our rescue and we all shook hands. Everyone was happy and I was very relieved to find myself once more on the ground with everything intact. Shortly afterwards we walked down to the bottom end of the strip and the District Commissioner performed the opening ceremony and cut the tape which had been hurriedly put across the strip. He recounted the story of how the strip had come to be made and how hard the local people had worked to get it ready. All this was true and as we walked slowly back up the strip I felt thankful that another hospital had been put on to the Flying Doctor network. As we approached the aircraft, an old lady dressed in skins came up to Father Staples and asked whether she could be introduced to the man who had brought in the 'Tin Bird'. She spoke in the vernacular so I could not understand what she said. I grasped her gnarled hands and gave them a good shake. She then proceeded to walk round the plane scrutinizing it carefully, finally coming back to the Father and saying:

'I can see the wings of this bird but where is the head?'

This final comment finished off the episode in the right vein. The take-off was easy as it was downhill and into the wind. We learnt from this experience that at certain times of the year when the wind was strong, we had to arrive before 10.00 a.m. or late in the evening. Another piece of bush flying lore had been gathered and tucked away into the communal memory of the Flying Doctor pilots and it stood us in good stead, but the real credit went to Father Staples and his helpers who had had the dream and the will to set out and accomplish it.

The more we thought about our problems the more it became clear that the key to the whole issue lay in better communications, and this is why in the early days we concentrated on putting in high-frequency radios to the peripheral hospitals so that we could have personal contact on a doctor to doctor or nurse to nurse basis. With a radio control in Nairobi, it became possible to render a growing number of services to these isolated hospitals in the bush and we were very grateful to the Nuffield Foundation when they helped us purchase the first twenty radios. They were placed at the hospitals which had least access to other forms of communication – in fact we started at the periphery and worked inwards. From the moment we installed the radios we sensed that this was going to play a very important part in our future endeavours. It telescoped the size of the problem and instead of having to go through operators, we could talk directly and immediately to each other. In future years I was constantly to be reminded of the effect the radio has on the morale of people working in the bush. It is a real lifeline. Being able to pick the brains of another medical man on a difficult case is comforting and often helpful; it shares the responsibility even on occasions when all we could say from the Nairobi control was 'there is nothing more to do, you have done everything possible'. Mission doctors have said to me, 'We know now that if one of our kids gets sick, we can get hold of you for immediate help.' This surely was what Mr Flynn was describing when he talked of the mantle of safety.

Very often a radio conversation can settle an issue without anyone having to move. In the past, on occasions, doctors had to travel hundreds of miles to get to a telephone or deliver a patient to a reference hospital. We have had some amusing and tricky situations over the radio network such as the time when a good mission doctor was putting a stainless steel nail down the narrow cavity of a man's leg which had been fractured, in order to immobilize the bones. The procedure can be a very good one but, as bad luck would have it on this occasion, the nail was somewhat large for the particular femur and, after getting it half in he could not get it any farther, and he could not get it out. In the circumstances and with inadequate tools any doctor might have found himself in the same predicament. Anyhow, this doctor left the theatre and kept his patient under anaesthesia and went to the radio to call us in Nairobi. After he explained the problem we scratched our heads and finally suggested that he should find a hacksaw in the carpenter's workshop, sterilize by boiling it in the instrument sterilizer and cut the nail off close to the bone, sew the wound up and we would come and fetch the patient and see what we could do. Forty minutes later the doctor came back on the radio to say he had successfully completed this task and the patient's condition was satisfactory. This man was picked up later by plane, returned to Nairobi, where the matter was sorted out with some difficulty, and a smaller nail inserted to hold the fracture.

I will give another example of the importance of radio communication.

Our radio engineer had recently been down at Haydom to install a high-frequency radio and he showed me on the map its position because it was my turn for the first surgical safari there. I took with me Rena Schweitzer, the daughter of Dr Albert Schweitzer, who was staying in Kenya for three weeks. She was repaying a visit which we had previously paid to Lambarene in the Gabon. We took off early and it was a clear, bright morning. I had worked out my course and felt reasonably happy about being able to find this mission. My estimate worked out at one hour and forty-five minutes' flying and a distance of two hundred and fifty miles from Nairobi.

Our route took us over some of the most spectacular country in Africa. It has always intrigued me that you only have to leave Nairobi thirty miles behind and you are back in prehistory, in country which has not been touched by man since the Creation. We crept under a layer of low stratus into the Rift Valley and left Lake Magadi on our starboard side. We crossed land which looked like the surface of the moon, dry, volcanic, ridged and desolate. Occasionally a herd of Maasai cattle could be seen straggling out from the manyatta where they had been incarcerated during the night. The dust rose into the air from their hooves and showed me the general direction of the wind. We flew on down past Shombole, the mountain which guards the northern shore of Lake Natron, out across this calm soda lake while we looked down at its surface of cracked white soda tinged blood red in places with ferric oxide. The clouds were mirrored on the surface of the lake and in places the reflection was so realistic that it was difficult to be sure whether we were not flying upside down. Then the scene changed as flocks of flamingoes began to fly out over the calm surface of the lake or sky, whichever it was. Here these amazing birds will nest at certain times, away from human interference. It has been calculated that there are three million of these birds going backwards and forwards between the lakes of the Rift Valley between Manyara and Hannington. Pelicans are down there too. On we sped over the arid country, climbing up the foothills of the Ngoro Ngoro crater, one of the great wonders of the world. We leave Ol Donyo Lengai on our port side as we start climbing to get over the high ground. This cone-like peak erupts every seven years and is the only active volcano in East Africa. Its sides are steep and covered with volcanic ash from a recent eruption which killed so much of the grazing and the wild animals too. I had flown over it during its active period and looked down into the narrow bubbling cauldron of red-hot lava. It would throw hot ash at least two thousand feet into the air above its crater edge.

Ngoro Ngoro was looking its best this morning as we passed just to starboard of it but close enough to see the flat floor of the crater with its lakes and quantities of game. I remembered going down into the crater before there was a road, and discovering this sanctuary which has since become well-known as one of the beauty spots of the world. We looked at the rim, which is sixty miles round, and the deep green forest which hides so many elephant and buffalo. As we cleared the high ground, Lake Eyasi lay below us, almost white in the sun. I had marked on my map the place where I thought we should come across its southern coast. I made for this small promontory so as to be sure I was on course when it came to finding Haydom Hospital. Half an hour later I came out over the mission and was secretly congratulating myself on my professional navigation. I circled round seeing a large cross on a hill and the various mission buildings. All was well except I could not see the airstrip. I decided to call up Dr Olsen, who was in charge at Haydom, and see what he had to say.

'Haydom, Haydom, do you read?' Silence. I tried again.

'Roger, Roger,' came Dr Olsen's cheery voice. 'Where are you?'

'Over your mission,' I said with confidence, 'but where is the airstrip?'

'But we cannot see or hear you,' said Dr Olsen.

My confidence began to ebb. After a long discussion we decided that I must be over Isansu, twenty-five miles to the west.

'Keep talking to me on the radio,' I said. 'Can you give me an idea of your exact position on the map? What relation has your hospital to Lake Eyasi?'

Dr Olsen finally went off to his office and got out a map. He drew a line on my instructions from the south-west corner of Lake Eyasi to Hanang, an 11,000-feet mountain to the south-east.

'Now which side of the line are you?' I asked.

'To the south and west of it,' he replied.

'OK,' I said. 'Can you please measure the distance along the line which will bring me out opposite Haydom.'

'Roger, I'll do that, wait a minute.' Well, as you know, you cannot wait in the air, you have to go somewhere. I was beginning to worry about my fuel and I wondered what Rena was thinking as we turned round yet again in the air.

'It's about thirty miles,' came Dr Olsen's voice.

'Roger,' I said. 'I shall proceed to the south-west corner of the lake and then point my plane at Hanang and fly for thirty miles, but do not leave the radio, please.' At the end of the lake I turned and looked for Hanang – there it was – I steered 145° and flew for twelve minutes. I noticed Dr Olsen's transmission was getting louder – that at least was some encouragement.

'Right,' I said, 'I have flown thirty miles. Where are you now?'

'Can you see an escarpment running in a southerly direction?'

'Yes,' I said, but without much conviction.

'Well, the mission is on the top of the escarpment by a hill covered in boulders.' A bright light suddenly caught my eye for a moment. What was that? Could it be the sun shining on a corrugated roof? Yes, it was, and now I could make out the mission buildings.

'The strip is not near the hospital, it is four miles away at the bottom of the escarpment. Oh, we can see you now.'

'Right,' I said, 'I've got you now. Have you put up a windsock?'

'Yes,' he said, 'it is near the south-west end.'

I did one low pass over the field to see what the surface looked like and then round again and made my run in. I was glad to be on the ground and was soon surrounded by hundreds of people who had never seen an aeroplane on the ground before. I got out and introduced Rena to Dr Olsen and we had a good laugh. I later found out that the radio engineer had marked the mission on the map twenty-five miles too far to the west. This restored my pride in my navigation but it also taught me a sharp lesson — never take anything for granted unless you have seen it yourself.

We were treated to generous Norwegian hospitality and Ole Olsen and I became firm friends, which we remain today.

As always at these remote places, I had an immense respect for the people who day after day follow their calling and un-complainingly put in a prodigious number of hours' work. They prove, if proof be necessary, that man is happy provided he has a dedication to his job and can fulfil himself doing something which his heart tells him is right. No one needs to be sorry for the solitary missionary families because they derive an inner satisfaction which compensates for all the sacrifices they make. I have never seen people who were more radiantly happy, confident and assured.

Without the contributions made by the missions medical care even today would be reduced by nearly 50 per cent in East Africa. This effort which started about a hundred years ago has largely gone unsung. Perhaps the impact has not been as great as it could have been because the Christian Church itself has been divided into so many different sects, which must have been as confusing to the African as it has been to the rest of the world. Nevertheless, the medical side of the mission effort has been a remarkable endeavour, both in dedication and hard work, often under tough and lonely conditions. To me the particular views and dogma of any one mission are not important, as I believe there are many roads which lead to the same goal. By and large the missionaries have set a high standard and a fine example. Perhaps they concentrated too much on curative medicine and on occasion used medical care as a tool for proselytizing, but, despite these and other criticisms, their record has been one of supreme achievement.

I find it easier to believe in a design and purpose in life rather than the opposite, which indicates that the whole of Creation is haphazard and meaningless. The intricacy of nature seems so astounding that it is difficult for me to believe it happened by chance. I have found, too, that most people whom I admire have a religious sense, even if they are not church-goers, and this is true not only of great men and women but also of people doing ordinary jobs. Convinced Christians usually manage to radiate a sense of conviction and often a happiness which goes with it. I have often noticed this among Christians of all types working in the bush in Africa. They have about them a certain authority and inner confidence which they can convey to others. Even their expressions help to tell the same story and give a meaning to their lives. Laurens van der Post in one of his books had this to say on the subject of meaning:

The real, the only crime out of which all evils came was a crime of meaning. It was the terrible invasion of meaningless- ness and a feeling of not belonging invading the awareness of man, that was the unique sickness of our day.

Many people find that the notion of a personal God is un- acceptable to them and that they cannot conceive of any God being interested in their petty affairs. That has not been my experience.

More than any subject, religion has had a major upheaval over the last few generations and many people would feel that it is largely discredited. More books are written on religion than any other subject, which at least shows that the controversy still rages and that answers are being sought now as always on the issue of 'what life is all about'. Through the ages Christianity has been held up as an ideal concept much admired in theory but little followed in practice. One of the main central themes of Christianity is the belief in life after death and perhaps the modern fear of death is due to the common inability to believe this tenet.

Society is troubled today by the ethical question of whether it is permissible to allow someone to die under certain conditions, when for one reason or another that person is living only a vegetable-type life artificially supported by modern medical tech- niques. You hear the expressions 'freedom to die' and 'being allowed to die with dignity'. A recent television programme examined this subject in depth and showed that there are many divergent opinions. In the issue of euthanasia the crux comes when the question is raised as to who has the right to decide. Many would answer, only God, and it is not possible or desirable for human beings to decide when a life should be brought to a close. Though fraught with many dangers, it is a problem which society must be forced to consider. I believe that keeping people alive artificially, when all hope has disappeared of a thinking existence, is wrong, and that it is not the job of the doctors to inflict this unnecessary prolongation of life.

In the end, religion is something you experience or you do not and intellectual argument always fails to produce the proof and only personal experience can convince. Within this enormous subject is it possible to express a faith which can mean anything to anyone else? In Hebrews we read:

Now faith is the substance of things hoped for, the evidence of things not seen.

Do we have to have everything proved to us through our finite intellects or can we sense truth in other ways? There is something in us described as conscience, which enables us to sense right from wrong. Is this merely something inculcated in us by our upbringing or is it more significant and more deeply buried in our nature?

It has been our privilege in AMREF to visit many different missions run by men and women of many nationalities. While AMREF itself is a non-sectarian organization, its staff are, of course, free to believe what they will. However, there can be few members of AMREF who have not been impressed by the work they have seen going on in the missions, and even if they do not always agree with what they see, they have developed a very healthy respect for the achievement.

It is always a delight to work in the missions because of their approach, which despises the trade unions' attitudes. No one watches the clock and if the work needs to go on late, nobody complains. I find this so refreshing in these days. Medicine cannot be dictated to by the clock and everyone works until the job is done. There is also no question of overtime. Apart from any other consideration, it leads to a good morale and team spirit, which cannot be gauged in material terms. Long may this way of tackling life continue to flourish in the missions.

6
A New Approach

It dawned on me slowly that only a small percentage of the inhabitants of the earth had access to medical care. I was staggered by a statement which a friend quoted to me that 50 per cent of the population of the world was born, lived and died without seeing a doctor. For someone brought up in the confines of a London medical school where each patient, it seemed, was seen by a number of doctors, this put a new complexion on the situation and I pondered on this thought and tried to put myself into the skin of an African living out in the bush. If you don't expect something, you don't miss it and this perhaps was why the rural dweller in Africa took life as it came, put up with its hardships, its lack of any basic health care, because he knew nothing better. It has always been a perplexing situation to realize that medical science today has a store of knowledge which, if applied, would make this world a happier place to live in, and yet we don't apply it, we go on doing more and more research because man's inquisitive mind will not let him rest until he knows it all. We can fly to the moon, but we can't begin to cover, even using aeroplanes, the remote parts of the globe, and so for the time being the unfortunate rural people of the developing world and many in the cities will miss out on the marvellous benefits that are available, and yet not available, to them. Professor J. K. Galbraith in a recent article hits the nail on the head

when he says that our western society 'has an appetite for
analysis but not for action'. It is as if simply stating the problem
automatically solves it. And so it is the lack of implementation
which dogs our feet every day in Africa. There are plans by the
score, conferences, workshops, seminars and all the rest of the
paraphernalia of modern planning, but the sad thing is that there
are very few people to implement the decisions of the planners
and so another report goes into the bottom drawer and is conveniently forgotten. This does not mean that planning is not
entirely necessary, but it is too uncomfortable to go out to where
the action is required; it means sacrificing some of the con-
veniences of modern life which we tend to take for granted.
Social amenities, schools and entertainment are missing and there
may be no electric light, insufficient water for a bath, too many
mosquitoes buzzing around and no air conditioning.

The graduates from our universities today shy away from the
job which needs to be done and often prefer to huddle with their
comrades in the ivory towers of our large cities discussing the
intricacies of some disease which is of no real consequence to
the overall health problem. It would be unfair to say that there
are no exceptions and it must be admitted that this unfortunate
situation is found all over the world.

It is a criticism of the medical profession today that it is
doctor- and hospital-oriented but not patient-oriented. The reputation of the profession and the high regard in which it was held by
the public are not quite the same today, and perhaps one of the
reasons is that the personal touch is missing. There are good
reasons for doctors to arrange for patients to see them by appoint-
ment in their offices but it is not the same thing as going to the
patient's home, getting to know the family and generally being
a friend and adviser. In the era of cost effectiveness this is one
of the things which has gone and many people must mourn its
passing. For a long time to come medical auxiliaries will be bearing the brunt of rural practice and in many ways they are better
suited to it.

As in all professions, experience is something you cannot buy,
and only slowly, as I learnt from my colleagues and from my own
mistakes, did I begin to understand some of the great health issues
which face us. They have very little to do with surgery, so it
took me a long time to grasp the real priorities. In Africa you

have to unlearn so many things which you learnt with such care in medical school. The situation is so different, as are the resources. The slavish copying of western methods and their applications to differing circumstances has led to a great deal of frustration, muddle and wrong priorities. In discussing what can be done in the circumstances which prevail today, I often ask people what they would do if they were suddenly to find themselves made Director of Medical Services of one of the developing countries of Africa. What would your priorities be? How would you spend your limited budget? Would you encourage family planning? Would you concentrate on preventive services or spend more on hospitals?

These and many other questions became the main ingredients of our discussions in AMREF. The diverse experiences of my senior colleagues all helped to mould a philosophy of medical care which we felt made sense under the restraints which were put on us by the lack of resources. We have come out strongly in favour of certain priorities and our views have been reinforced by our experience in other African countries where our advice has been sought from time to time.

It is helpful to know some of the basic statistics without which no real planning can begin. Often accurate statistics are not available but death rates and birth rates are better known now that a number of national censuses have been held. Kenya has a population of thirteen million and some two dollars per head to spend on health per year. Although the doctor-patient ratio overall is higher than in many African countries, the distribution is very uneven and most of these doctors work in the larger towns. At the present time there are sixty medical officers at district level for the whole of Kenya, but the mission doctors help to swell the numbers and often man the most peripheral rural hospitals. In fact the doctor-patient ratio is not very useful as a statistic and at times most misleading, because it is necessary to know many other factors concerning the availability of medical auxiliaries and nurses to get a balanced picture.

How do you get the best value for your money when dealing with health? This was the sort of question which I was asking myself all the time. Unfortunately for the individual, clinical medicine and hospitals are the most expensive forms of treatment and it is easy to allow far too high a proportion of the budget to be spent on those items. Political pressures tend to reinforce this aspect. Approximately 1 per cent of the population go through hospitals a year. What are we going to do about the 99 per cent? Surely they deserve some consideration. Of this 99 per cent almost half will be children under the age of fifteen. Here is one priority. Treat the children. Preventive measures such as vaccinations must come high up the list, for not only is prevention better than cure but it is also ten times cheaper. The so-called developed world is now being overtaken by a crisis in its curative services because the cost is escalating to a frightening extent and no one wants to be the first to call a halt, though that day must come.

AMREF has at times helped in the control of epidemic disease, and one incident comes to mind when we were asked by the Regional Medical Officer in Arusha in Northern Tanzania to fly to Dar-es-Salaam and collect many thousands of tablets of sulpha-methazine which he wanted urgently to give to seven thousand people who were in the immediate vicinity of an outbreak of pneumonic plague. The first case had been admitted to Mbulu district hospital to the west of Arusha and had died, as did two of the nursing staff who had looked after this patient. The medical officer fortunately made and confirmed the correct diagnosis. I set off for Dar-es-Salaam in a Piper Aztec aircraft to obtain as many of the required tablets as I could fit into this twin-engined machine. I remember arriving at the central Medical Stores in the capital and emptying the contents of small tins of sulphametha-zine into old but clean four-gallon petrol tins in order to save space in the aircraft and make it easier to pack. This operation seemed to take a long time in the heat of Dar-es-Salaam and it was some hours before I could head for Arusha with an over-loaded plane which flew through the air like a pregnant duck. It was very tail-heavy and this reduced my speed, but the journey was uneventful and when I arrived at Arusha a smaller plane of the Flying Doctor Service was ready at the airfield to ferry the drugs in relays into the small, recently constructed airstrip at Mbulu. In a short time the drugs were efficiently distributed to the people at risk in the district and in the end only a total of seven cases, including the first three, were struck down by this very virulent disease.

On another occasion we were asked to consider inoculating the whole population of the Kilimanjaro region against polio. There had been one hundred and seventy-seven cases there and the population were greatly concerned for their children. Three months of careful preparation took place in explaining to the people what had to be done and setting up the necessary operation. The Council of the Chagga people in Moshi gave their full co-operation and all the various authorities were instructed about the coming campaign. We even took children who had become paralysed with the disease to demonstrate to the parents what could happen to their children if they did not bring them for inoculation. Leaflets were distributed and the information campaign began to infiltrate the farthest corners of the Kilimanjaro district. In the meantime a generous company in the USA donated enough vaccine to inoculate four hundred thousand young people under the age of twenty-one. This was the number which we calculated needed to be inoculated. Arrangements were made to fly this vaccine, carefully refrigerated, from the USA and get it into local refrigerators which had been installed at strategic places on the mountain. Finally the great day came and the people started lining up at sixty centres to receive the vaccine on a piece of sugar. The turnout was almost 100 per cent and the campaign successful beyond our wildest dreams. No more cases of polio occurred but we had to think of the follow-up and how these inoculations could be continued in order to produce a lasting effect in safeguarding the growing generation.

It is a simple calculation to work out in rough terms what treating one hundred and seventy-seven children with polio can involve. Firstly there is the initial period in hospital where the most acute cases will die, and all the expense involved in the nursing care. Then there are the years ahead which will be punctuated by repeated return visits to hospital for orthopaedic operations, physiotherapy, splints and the rest of the armamentarium of modern curative medicine. Then there is the incalculable cost in crippled lives which must be taken into consideration in the final tally. This, more than any other incident, convinced me where the priorities must be. It was abundantly clear.

Public health measures such as the providing of clean water supplies are another priority and could prevent untold quantities of water-borne disease, which it is reckoned in some areas amounts to 50 per cent of all diseases. It is a common experience to visit a hospital at the top of a hill and see expensive drugs such as antibiotics being dispensed to deal with dysenteries and such-like diseases. If you take the trouble to go to the bottom of the hill and inspect where the water supply comes from you will often readily appreciate why the antibiotics have to be dispensed in such quantities. Clearly the priority is to clean up the water supply but this will be a major undertaking which some Governments in Africa are just beginning to tackle.

At times local beliefs and customs interfere with the health of the people. There are certain areas proving intransigent to the control of cholera. Local tradition holds that when someone dies relatives must converge for the funeral and each one has to kiss or touch the body before it is buried. Obviously this custom was a source of the spread of cholera and its persistence.

Yet another priority in the health field with which few would disagree is training. It is better to train ten people to do your job than work ten times as hard yourself. AMREF is now busy helping to run courses for medical auxiliaries and produce manuals to fill the reading gap for them. Building up a small library of appropriate books for those working in the bush has become a central theme for us. At the present time Kenya has some eight hundred Clinical Officers; these men bear the brunt of the clinical load all over the country and without them doctors would be totally swamped. They help to screen the patients so that the doctor can see those patients which really require his particular skills. They receive a four-year training and their horizons are adjusted to the local scene.

Although everyone will agree that training has a high priority there is much more divergence of opinion as to what this training should include. We need to train people to do the job which is there to be done. This would sound simple enough, but in fact it is not so easy. Medical students tend to become involved in the minutiae of clinical care and the rare case has a fascination far beyond its importance. Dr H. Mahler, Director General of the World Health Organization, recently had this to say on the subject of Medical Schools:

Most of the world's medical schools prepare doctors, not to care for the health of the people, but instead for medical practice that is blind to anything but disease and the technology for dealing with it; a technology involving astronomical and ever-increasing prices, directed towards fewer and fewer people who are often selected not so much by social clan or wealth as by medical technology itself, and frequently focused on persons in the final stages of life. They prepare doctors to deal with rare cases which are hardly ever encountered, rather than with the common health problems of the community; for cure rather than for care. They tend to forget that technical solutions must respond to social goals, not dictate them. Medical practice has become almost synonymous with curative medicine and doctors are trained predominantly to look at episodes of disease, paying little or no heed to the whole man, and to his interaction with society.*

This whole subject is being scrutinized at many levels now and out of it must come a more realistic and appropriate policy. It is the social aspects of poverty and ignorance which need to be changed before medical services can really make the impact they should.

WHO and national Governments of the third world are now stressing the importance of training of the 'Community Health Worker' to be the first line of defence. He will be the man or woman chosen by the village to receive a short course in the basics of environmental health which will include supervising water supplies, rural sanitation, refuse disposal, housing, vermin and pest control, nutrition, care of food, health education and assisting with immunization campaigns. He will also be taught to treat the ten more common local diseases in an empirical fashion. It has been shown in several areas of the world that a man with common sense and who is trusted by his community can make a vital contribution to health at village level even if he has only a primary education.

In the Southern Sudan AMREF has been entrusted with the task of the training of the teachers for this new cadre, the Community Health Worker, and the first students are coming in for their courses which will last for nine months. As there are many thousands of villages, it will grow into a major programme over the coming years.

It is at this grass-roots level that there is much to be done

---

* From an address (originally in French) given by Dr H. Mahler, Director-General of the World Health Organization, at the centenary celebration of the Faculty of Medicine of the University of Geneva, in Geneva on 28 October 1976: *Tomorrow's Medicine and Tomorrow's Doctors.*

which doctors and hospitals alone will never be able to do. Supervision of these men and women in their villages is essential if standards are to be maintained, and this can best be done by those who taught them in the first place. Refresher courses will help to maintain morale and stimulate interest with new ideas.

The philosophy of priorities which I have outlined is gaining acceptance at many levels, but there is still a hard core of resistance in the medical profession who perhaps feel that the emphasis on training auxiliaries is a threat to their own position.

The subject of health education can prove to be of overwhelming importance to the individual and can be achieved at very little cost. It is, however, a subject fraught with misunderstandings. The most important advances in health lie in influencing the behaviour of people, and this is a slow battle which will only be won yard by yard. For instance I have had to deal with severe burns in people of all ages in Africa. Babies crawl into the fire which is kept burning on the floor of the hut, or pull an inviting-looking saucepan off the fire, scalding themselves in so doing. Some of the worst burns, however, are those in epileptics who fall into the fire during a fit, and as the disease is believed to be contagious at this stage no one will pull them out or go to their aid and they burn most terribly. Both these examples could be eliminated from the list of medical problems if education in these matters could alter behaviour patterns. What can you do in your own home to safeguard your health and the health of your family? This subject is difficult to teach and prejudices abound, but over the last twenty years small areas of progress can now be seen. It is not only a problem for developing countries, it is universal.

We have learnt that individual person-to-person contact is the best way of persuasion and that posters, slides and other visual aids are sadly disappointing when dealing with people who are illiterate and not used to looking at screens. The old story of the mosquito epitomises what I am trying to say. A nurse on my staff was lecturing on malaria to a group of tribesmen. She threw a picture on a screen which showed a greatly magnified mosquito, and went on to talk about the transmission of malaria from the mosquito to man. At the end of the lecture a man stood up to say that malaria could not be a problem to them because they didn't have mosquitoes that size! We may laugh but really it was quite a logical statement. Without being accustomed to the habit of perspective and deliberate magnification for purposes of explanation, it is quite strange to be confronted with this type of visual education and it is not surprising that such incidents occur. It was only when the head of our Health Education department wrote a book on this subject that I began to understand the difficulties involved in explaining things to people of another culture. I am sure that many people are blissfully ignorant that their words of wisdom and beautiful slides may be interpreted in a very different way from what was intended. The final error is to think that people, whose reactions are different because of different experience, are stupid. Far from it; they may be very intelligent but living in a different idiom.

As people become more aware of what they can do to protect their own health in the home, so a fitter generation will evolve. It is already happening but it is painfully slow. Talks on the radio or television are an additional source of information to the general public and this again slowly has an effect on attitudes and finally behaviour. Health or the lack of it is a complex subject and over-simplification does not help. The real underlying problems must be brought into the open and viewed in their relation to social development in other spheres.

Of all paramedical subjects family planning is still the most controversial, and it would be shirking the issue not to mention it. The world population is doubling now every twenty-five years or so. The figures are terrifying and the medical profession is often accused of making the situation worse by keeping more people alive. This is a very superficial way of looking at the problem. It is basically a social issue and not a medical one. If given the sanction of society the medical profession can readily keep the birth rate down. Is our society ready to do this? Is legal compulsion going to be necessary? I am told that population growth has been levelled out in China and Japan. It is simply not fashionable to have more than two children per family and it is a disgrace not to comply with the Government edict while abortion is freely available.

In western countries the population growth started to level off long before the pill. Doubtless modern contraceptive methods have made it easier but the economic arguments have been strong and compelling and these in time will also be persuasive forces in the developing countries. Of one thing I am sure – that the ordinary peasant woman in Africa is not going to listen much to family-planning propaganda until more of her children live. Children in tribal life are a source of help and wealth and also provide care for their parents in their old age when there is no old age pension. Infant mortality is still very high in many areas and so a woman may feel she has to have ten children to be sure she will be left with four living ones. We can hardly blame her. None of this argument is intended to deny the supreme importance of this question, as it could be said to be the most important health problem of all. It is a perfectly soluble problem once society as a whole is ready and prepared to do what is necessary. If we are going to allow it to be dealt with without compulsion, then a new discipline will be required and a rapid extension of education on all aspects of this vital issue. If we insist on our freedom to choose in these matters, which is the way, perhaps, the democracies would prefer, then we had better choose quickly and wisely now.

AMREF brings this subject into the wider concept of health education and it is taught as part of maternal and child health, which is where it belongs.

During the early pioneering days of AMREF we thought we should experiment with using mobile vans to bring medicine in its various forms to people where there were as yet no static services, while radios and light aircraft were used to help supply these units and keep them in touch with the outside world. Unless they are very carefully administered and run these units can be expensive and wasteful.

I remember an occasion when I went to seek permission from the Ministry of Health to take a mobile unit up to Turkana in the north-western desert area of Kenya. Fired by enthusiasm but not yet fully aware of the difficulties I sat down in the Director of Medical Services' office and asked whether a unit could be operated out of Lodwar. The then Director, and this was in the colonial days, said to me, 'You know, Michael, you will go up there and do your work and then you'll come back and tell me there are a lot of sick Turkana. We know that already and we haven't got the resources to cover that vast area.' He looked at me in a fatherly fashion with a twinkle in his eye.

'You know, sir,' I said, 'that this is one of the reasons we started AMREF, to complement and supplement the existing services.'

'Well, I'm sorry,' he said, 'for the time being the answer is NO.'

So that was it. I have since got used to dealing with the Civil Service mind. I realized that it was so much easier to say no because if you said yes this would mean a lot more work, but in all fairness I knew that the medical services were fully stretched. Their policy was a simple one and basically it was founded on some incontrovertible facts such as the size of the health budget and the personnel available to carry out the service.

We experimented with different types of mobile units and rapidly learnt some vital factors in the game. We discovered that large heavy units, even with four-wheel drive, become a liability in the rains when they are apt to sink up to their axles in mud. Sophisticated interiors were also a potential menace as the unit was shaken about on the pot-holed country roads and things began to break up and break down! Simplicity and rugged construction were necessities if the vehicle was to stand up to the hammering it would inevitably get. Many very good companies have designed some excellent mobile units which have done good work in the USA and Europe, but if this type of vehicle is tried on African roads they break down and finally come to be used as chicken houses or stores at the side of the road where they have come to grief. So we settled on the light truck, the Land-Rover or the Toyota Land Cruisers. They were less expensive to run, more flexible on the job and stood up far better to the conditions.

It is still difficult to come up with an acceptable list of priorities where curative medicine is concerned, for stern decisions have to be taken which do not face the doctor in places more extensively provided with medical facilities. I remember in the very early days in Africa, on a visit to the West Coast, hearing an orthopaedic surgeon refuse over the radio to admit a case of a fractured spine to his paraplegic unit. He already had every bed full and only enough staff to deal with those he had, as each patient required two hours a day of individual nursing. He knew, as we knew who heard him, that this decision meant the man would die, but in the circumstances which rigidly and starkly dictated the terms in which he could practise medicine, he had no alternative.

Our mobile units staff are faced with such decisions, though they also have the reward of seeing patients return to them month after month and see them improve and get well. We have learnt that regularity in visiting places has helped the units to become accepted and gain the confidence and co-operation of the people. I have seen our teams set up their clinic to all appearances in the open desert, under some spreading thorn tree through which the wind whistles, taking all important pieces of paper, such as patients' notes, with it. The dust, too, would be swirled about by the wind, penetrate surgical dressings and every attempt at surgical technique. Slowly a brown figure would emerge from the empty landscape and squat beside the unit until finally a crowd had gathered with many women and children among them. The people somehow knew the time and place of the arrival of the unit even though they measured time by the phases of the moon, and it was important to them that it would also be there the following month.

We have been most fortunate in having some very dedicated staff who have, over the years, ironed out many of the problems. They know what can be done and what cannot be done by the mobile method. Careful planning, regular visits, proper equipment and learning to be entirely self-supporting are all essential ingredients. And even when you think that you have evolved a foolproof system, exciting things can still happen. Wild animals have succeeded in getting the staff of a mobile unit up into the trees for safety, and flash floods have caused alarming moments of involuntary swimming and destruction of equipment. But between these infrequent but frightening episodes, a routine has been hammered out of experience, and medical care brought to nomadic areas in a way which is understood, appreciated and has a lasting impact.

I have set out some of the factors in this approach to medicine in the developing countries because it seemed to me that it needed some explanation and indeed justification. It was not a case of settling for the second best but an attempt to provide medical care in an appropriate way for the rural population with people who were trained to improvise and work within the many restraints imposed by both the economy and the geography. We felt that the methods had to be tailor-fitted to the actual prevailing situation so that the frontiers of medicine could be pushed out into the really needy places where such a high proportion of the population lived. What we have been able to do is only a drop in the ocean but maybe it will help to stimulate others, and in the end a multiplication effect may be seen. The day will come when static services alone are adequate to cope with the rural peoples and sufficient medical teams will be available. Other facilities will grow alongside the medical ones, and schools, housing, water supplies and other amenities will become more abundant as community development proceeds; but this is likely to take several generations and in the meantime the mobile approach has its advantages if co-ordinated within the overall policies. While concentrating on the rural areas for the time being, it is menacingly clear that enormous problems abound in the urban areas, and as the populations of the cities of the developing world are increasing sharply, new approaches in medical care will be called for to cope with the urban poor.

7
Surgery in the Bush

In any Flying Doctor Service it is essential for bush doctors and pilots to be able to improvise. However hard you try it is difficult to foresee and bring everything which you may require to deal with a host of different medical and surgical problems. Let one example suffice.

I was down in Western Tanzania near Lake Tanganyika doing a formidable list of operation cases. As so often happens the pathology is far advanced and many patients report late about their ills. A man came in with the story of a fall four months before – he had been unable to walk since but had hobbled about hanging on to one long pole which he used as a crutch. Examination revealed that he had a dislocated hip and X-rays showed that the head of the femur had ridden up a long way on to the side of his pelvis. I decided, perhaps unwisely, to try and reduce the dislocation by open operation. Starting late in the evening after a whole day in the theatre, I exposed the head of the femur, cleared out the soft tissue lying in the socket into which the head must go, and then, with three strong fellows pulling on the leg, I struggled to reduce the dislocation. After a fearsome tug-of-war it became very obvious to us all that we were making little or no progress. I went and sat down on a stool to think what to do next; everyone was tired but determined not to admit defeat. The problem is a difficult one even in perfect circumstances with every modern surgical invention to hand, but I did not have strong enough bone holders and bone levers to get sufficient purchase. A rare flash of genius came to me: why not use a tyre lever – had they got one? Go and look in the Land-Rover. A theatre assistant came back triumphant, wielding a large, dirty tyre lever. Galvanized into action, I took off my gown and gloves and called for some emery paper. I washed the tyre lever, getting off the grease, gave it a good scrub and then set to to rub away the rust from the surface. Half an hour later the lever was carefully sterilized and I re-scrubbed to join battle once again. With the head of the femur lying on the inside of the tyre lever I was able to slowly ease it towards its proper home. We had about three inches to go – slowly but surely, with the three good men and true pulling on the leg, we began to see that victory was within reach and then suddenly there was a loud clunk as the head snapped back into its socket. We closed the wound and went off at about eleven o'clock to what we felt was a well-earned supper. In the morning we X-rayed the patient just to check all was well. The wound healed slowly; the patient in time got back on his feet, and although he limps a little he has a serviceable hip.

As our struggles went on I was intrigued day by day by certain traits in the African character, particularly his stoicism and his sense of humour. Examples of these characteristics abound and kept coming my way and helped to mould my ideas, so I recount a few here, as they formed the background to much that happened.

The fatalism and courageous acceptance of life were epitomized for me by a Turkana patient whom I saw on a ward round at Kakuma, near the Sudan border. The sisters showed me a man who had a horrifying condition of his hands. It transpired that this man, who was a kind of witch doctor, had been condemned for putting a spell on a certain village. He was taken out into the desert and in the blazing sun tied to a stake by thongs round both his wrists. He was left there without food or water. Ten days later, one of his sons returned to the village from a journey and heard the fate of his father. He went straight out into the desert and found his father still alive. In trying to free himself he had stripped all the flesh off both hands. He had managed to keep off the hyenas and vultures and survived the appalling thirst which must have attacked him. The son released his father and helped the old man walk back to the hospital, a distance of many miles. When I heard this story I found it hard to believe. But even if the time interval had been exaggerated, it was an extraordinary feat of endurance. One arm had to be amputated and a small remnant of the other hand was saved. He never complained and when his wounds healed he returned home.

I could recount many stories of similar heroism and endurance. I do not believe that the African patient feels less pain than a white man; he is more used to it and is able to accept it, as the white man did before the days of anaesthetics. You only have to read the account of Admiral Nelson and the way in which he withstood his many wounds to realize that men of that era and before were just as unflinching and stoical.

This quality in the African patient makes him a great deal easier to look after. He also seems on occasions to have a remarkable power of recovery. I was doing an out-patient clinic in the Kenyatta National Hospital one day when a friend of mine brought a Maasai moran, a warrior, in to see me.

'Michael,' he said, 'please take a look at this chap. I picked him up out in Maasailand and this is his story. Four months ago he was involved in a tribal battle with another clan of Maasai. He is the chief moran and on this occasion he was leading five hundred men against a thousand of the opposing clan. It was over the old problem of grazing. This man was speared through the thigh, high up, just below the crease of the buttock. Since then he has been limping around Maasailand and has developed some horrible sores on the sole of his foot. Can you please help him?'

I asked the Maasai warrior, who was a particularly fine specimen of manhood, to sit down, and I bent forward to pick up his foot. He had two deep ulcers on the sole of the foot which were infected and discharging. As I went on to examine him and watch him walk it was not difficult to discern that he had an injury involving his sciatic nerve. He dragged his leg, had a severe foot drop and had virtually no sensation on the back of his leg and foot.

I told my friend that I did not hold out much hope for recovery in this leg and that amputation might be the only possible outcome. However, I told him I would admit the Maasai, explore his wound and see what could be done to the sciatic nerve. He was an incongruous sight in the ward, as he was dressed as a Maasai warrior, covered in red ochre and his hair in a mud pack.

He bore the teasing and laughter of his fellow patients with disdain and dignity. A few days later, after we had had time to clean up the ulcers and prepare him for the operation, I took him to the operating theatre to explore his wound. Nerve fibres recover at about one millimetre per day, so a wound involving the sciatic nerve at the top of the thigh in a tall man will take eighteen months to recover if all goes well. I had given my friend this pessimistic prognosis.

After the anaesthetic had been given I placed the Maasai on his front and explored the wound made by the spear. After a short time I came on the sciatic nerve; seven-eighths of it had been severed. I was depressed by what I saw but determined to try and suture the nerve. I bent up his knee till his heel was above the wound and I released a long section of the nerve so that I could get the ends together without tension. The sciatic nerve is a mixed nerve, which means it has both motor and sensory fibres in it. To get a reasonable chance of any recovery this nerve had to be sutured so that there was no twisting on its axis. It was as thick as my index finger and badly scarred. I cut away almost half an inch of nerve on either side, including the remaining one-eighth which was still attached, though found to be mainly scar tissue. I approximated the ends with some difficulty and closed the wound. I then put him in plaster with his knee fully flexed. He lay on his front in bed in this rather undignified position. I reported to my friend that in my opinion he was most unlikely to get any recovery. After three weeks I extended his knee a little and replastered it. After six weeks he was over on his back and having physiotherapy. His recovery was, in fact, dramatic. I could not account for it and to this day it seems like a tall story. After four months he was walking quite well. His ulcers had healed and sensation had largely returned. He has resumed his ordinary life and his only residual defect is a slight foot drop which has never fully recovered. He walks twenty miles a day. How did this man's nerve recover at over four times the speed it normally does? I don't know, but I do know that he is walking about Maasailand and my friend is my witness. He was supremely fit at the time of his injury, which must have been a factor in his favour, but otherwise the matter remains a mystery. This type of case is an encouragement and helps one endure the many failures.

I have mentioned the African's sense of humour. It is an endearing quality. So often tense situations have been mollified by his ability to see the funny side of things and I have been so grateful many times for this valuable attribute.

On one occasion I was doing a safari in the area south of Nairobi with an old friend and patient of mine. Although retired he had been the doyen of the professional hunters and had taken out many VIPs in his day. He had kindly consented to accompany us and we were inducted into that marvellous life which is inherent in the word 'safari'. Life suddenly seems much more simple and the pleasures of good company, magnificent scenery and wild game make an exhilarating mixture. It is round the camp fire that many people have felt the healing qualities of the wild. The African night noises, the crackle of the fire, the cool air, are all inducive to real relaxation. We were even spoilt by having a canvas bath and hot water and I know no feeling more comforting than washing off the dust of the day, putting on a pair of pyjamas and dressing-gown and sitting, glass in hand, around the fire.

I have never been much interested in shooting big game and really we were only shooting for the pot. On the last few days of the safari I was told that our African staff would much appreciate being able to take some meat home. This seemed to me a reasonable request. They were a jolly crew of Wakamba and were well trained to safari life. We set off one morning to hunt for buffalo and though we saw some at great distance, we never got close enough for a shot. However, the next day, after a long and bumpy trek around the bushes, we began to see quite a large number of buffalo.

While inspecting my gun and seeing that I was properly prepared, a large buffalo emerged from the bushes and ran obliquely across me about seventy yards away. With some difficulty I got my gun loaded and fired at this huge beast, being careful to lead him a little as he was moving quite fast. I heard the thud of the bullet as it hit, but the buffalo did not hesitate or appear to be badly hit. He ran a hundred and twenty yards and then suddenly collapsed. I remember being amazed at the vitality of these creatures, when I eventually found out that the bullet had entered his chest and gone through the aorta, the largest artery in the body, as it came off the heart. The Africans were absolutely delighted with this good fortune and insisted that a photograph should be taken, *Tatler* style, with me, the intrepid hunter, standing on the fallen corpse. All was prepared and I stood on the buffalo's chest holding my gun and looking rather foolish.

As the photo was about to be taken the buffalo gave a tremendous jerk. I was seen doing a hundred yards in Olympic time in search of a small tree which I had spied. When I got there I desperately tried to force my large frame up through the thorns. At that moment I turned round to see how close the buffalo was behind me. The sight which met my eyes was not what I had expected. The buffalo appeared to be lying in the same position as before its reflex death spasm, and the Africans were rolling on the ground howling with laughter. They laughed till they cried, and until the last minute of the safari any reference to this undignified performance produced immediate paroxysms of mirth. The safari ended in an atmosphere of great friendliness and often since that day I have been warmed by the infectious good humour of African colleagues and friends. It goes a long way to ease the racial tensions which sometimes appear so suddenly. Laughter can disperse these quicker than other remedies.

Yes, we need to be made ridiculous from time to time. We desperately need this ingredient of humour to maintain our humanity and understand the human predicament. The African shares these moments to the full. I remember another ridiculous situation which occurred while taking part in a motor-car rally with Robin, who was extraordinarily adept at the art of moving along roads at prodigious speeds. I was his navigator and my main occupation was concentrated most of the time on getting him to take his right foot off the accelerator. In this rally we were doing rather well. As usual, my family and Robin's were manning the route and doing all they could to assist with our well-being. My son-in-law's father, in a moment of great generosity, threw into the rally car a bunch of bananas while I was out of the car getting our card signed at a control point. I was in such a hurry to get back to the car that I jumped in and unwittingly sat on the bunch of bananas. I was so concerned with the route that I didn't consciously appreciate what was going on below me. I think I remember beginning to feel that my bottom was getting chilly but I was so engaged on doing my job that it didn't really register. When we got to the finish, fortunately in an honoured position, we were met by many members of the family. I got out of the car cheered by a large African crowd and I was beginning to feel like a hero until one of my irreverent nephews sang out, 'Look at Uncle Mike.' The cat was out of the bag. The seat of my trousers was covered in squashed bananas. It was a riot; dignity vanished and I was left to scrape off this revolting mess, much to the amusement of the onlookers. The African crowd were delighted.

It is often said that Africans are lazy, but like most generalizations it is less than a half truth. I believe that the reason for laziness is often poor health. Some years ago we did a random sample of the blood picture of three thousand people from Lake Victoria to the Coast and found that the average haemoglobin was 52 per cent of normal. With this amount of anaemia it is not surprising that a man cannot complete a full day's work. Most of us wouldn't undertake to start.

Yet it would be stupid to pretend that a multi-racial society is an easy one in which to live. It needs a lot of give and take, the ability to laugh at oneself as well as at others, and a real desire to scale the racial barriers and like what you find on the other side. It is a situation constantly inflamed by prejudice and ignorance on all sides, and it is no good denying that it is the most explosive political issue of our day.

I have noticed that, apart from the African character, the African continent gives a different dimension to the work out here. For instance, flying up to Wajir in the north-eastern desert of Kenya is an especially romantic journey, as the green of the Highlands gives way gradually to the colours of the encroaching desert; Mount Kenya with its forest and glaciers fades gradually into the background while the Tana River curls away to the east. It is a perfect example of how altitude and rainfall are responsible for the changing scene below.

The light began to fade and I was beginning to reprimand myself for leaving our departure from Nairobi so late, but I had the Wajir beacon to steer by and this comforting fact prevented me from being too alarmed. I had left the road as it swings out to the east through Mado-Gashi, so I was west of Habaswein according to my calculations and about sixty miles from Wajir. It was half past six and at this precise moment the needle on my

ADF began to wander and I realized after a few seconds of thought that the beacon had been turned off in Wajir. Now I was going to have to think very hard to avoid having to make a forced landing in the fading light, somewhere in the desert below.

The sixty miles would take me twenty-four minutes at 150 m.p.h, which would bring me into Wajir at five minutes to seven when it would be almost completely dark. I was at 9500 feet and I reckoned I could save a few precious minutes if I started a gradual descent which would put up my speed. I knew or thought I knew that I was west of the main road and that if I steered a little more to the east I was bound to hit it, and I would then be able to follow it till I saw the lights of Wajir. The fading light began to play tricks with my imagination, as I was now worried and began to see things which were not there. I was not sure that I would be able to see the road and therefore might cross it without knowing and carry on into the desert and miss Wajir. This disquieting time did not last long, but long enough to teach me another sharp lesson. I spotted the road and flew on, keeping it carefully in my vision, and before long I saw the lights ahead and my troubles were over.

Mark, our eldest son, was waiting at the airstrip and we soon unloaded the plane and were heading towards his home in his Toyota Land Cruiser. Mark was the medical officer at Wajir and had an enormous district to cover. He was in his element and the medical king of all he surveyed. His quiet reflective personality coped well with the loneliness of his remote station, and his inner resources carried him serenely through his work which was varied, interesting and yet demanding. His staff held him in high respect and during his time there he was able to install running water in the hospital for the first time and also electric light, though the generator had a habit of playing up. He kept a record of all the tuberculosis patients he had seen, because the disease had affected the population in almost epidemic proportions and was perhaps the most important scourge with which he had to deal.

On the following day we started early in the theatre and saw a number of patients in the wards between operations. The sun went down after a long day, the breeze dropped, but the heat in the theatre seemed to be stifling.

The staff had worked willingly even when my temper began to shorten as I struggled to finish the last case. I was tired and was working slowly to sew up the last incision. As always on these occasions the thread began to break because I pulled too hard. I dropped the needle-holder on the floor. The generator failed, which meant pressure-lamps and a torch instead. Insects had invaded the theatre and fluttered around making a mockery of our sterile techniques. At last it was over; stalwart men came in with a stretcher and the last human bundle was carried off to the ward. It would take a time before he was round from the anaesthetic – a blissful time when consciousness was suppressed and with it the pain and discomfort of the operation.

I went back to the house, took off my operating pyjamas, which were stained with sweat and blood, and allowed the trickle of rainwater from the home-made shower to cool and cleanse me. Somewhat restored, I climbed up the steps on to the flat roof to sample the night air and gaze up at the canopy of heaven above. Wajir produces wonderful clear skies and with Mark's telescope we probed some of the secrets of the night. The stars forming the constellations are so many million light years away from each other that only to us, looking from earth, do they appear to form some sort of pattern. The telescope magnified seventy-five times and we spent a half-hour looking at the Pleiades.

The Pleiades are close to Taurus the Bull and look like a group of very faint stars. Through the telescope we could distinguish six individual stars. Apparently all those stars are travelling together through space. Aldebaran could be seen close by and is the brightest star in the constellation Taurus and has an orange colour.

Then I felt compelled to look at Andromeda and tried to recall the mythology in which she was involved. This unlucky lady, an Ethiopian princess, the daughter of Cepheus the King, was fastened to a rock by Poseidon for a whale to devour but was finally rescued by Perseus, her next-door neighbour in the universe. Her mother was Cassiopeia, also seen in the same part of the sky, shaped like a large W. Perseus carried off the beautiful Andromeda on his winged horse, Pegasus, after slaying the whale. The wing is fixed to the horse's rump. This is perhaps poor aerodynamic design but we can forgive Pegasus for this because with one blow of his hoof he created the fountain Hippocene, the source of poetic inspiration.

The depth of the universe is really inconceivable and you can get lost in it as you can when flying at night. The sky at night can be seen as a beautiful tapestry, but once you try to understand its size and meaning you are in a different dimension. You are forced to think about the design and purpose of it all. Your mind starts enquiring about why is the earth the only planet on which there is human life as we know it. Is this true? Are there going to be other stars or planets on which some kind of life is possible? After a time you can almost sense the movement of the earth through space and then at last your finite mind gives up the struggle of challenging the infinite and you are back on the roof at Wajir and thinking about the mundane matters of your terrestial existence. Fortunately in some ways, our minds have only a limited scope, and although some are gifted with great powers of imagination, who at the beginning of the century could really have forecast what was going to happen by 1978? Perhaps H. G. Wells and Jules Verne and a few others could score some marks here, but the acceleration of knowledge over this period of time has been totally beyond what we ordinary mortals could have conceived in our wildest dreams. Many books have been written recently on this phenomenon and they contain some sobering thoughts about our predicament.

What is referred to as the 'rat race' today has assumed terrifying proportions. It is difficult for anyone to remain serene and content in the kaleidoscopic conditions of modern life. It becomes increasingly difficult to hold on to your own soul and know who you are, because the battering of new stimuli turns you into a neurotic pulp worn out by trying to respond to so many distracting forces. This is why our age is so rootless and beset with such hideous alternatives. Our minds and spirits have not been able to cope with the acceleration. In the last thirty years human knowledge has doubled in volume, which means that more has been discovered in the last thirty years than in the whole of history before that time. No wonder we are confused; no wonder our mental institutions can no longer cope with the human breakdown which is occurring. Never before has life been so confronted with total destruction. To get relief from this overwhelming feeling of imminent doom, various tranquillizers have been resorted to and the consumption of drugs and alcohol has escalated to an alarming degree. Are we possessed like the lemmings?

Something inside us rejects this total catastrophic forecast for our future and yet it is most puzzling to define. There are a few hopeful signs that, as man has approached the brink, he has begun to realize where his present policies are leading him. The concern for the environment, for the conservation of animal life, for the control of energy and for the plight of the third world, are all matters which at last are receiving urgent attention. This is something, some ray of hope in a darkening scene that man is conscious of how little time there is left in which to take decisive action.

And yet I feel that really the only hope is for man's spirit to grow as fast as his scientific knowledge. The spirit has been left behind, ignored, trampled on and denied. We do this at our peril. Only when man turns back to the inner resources of his being is he going to be able to find the real ingredients which he needs to stay the course and to find his own salvation. Why is there this sudden fashion for yoga? It is because man is desperately seeking some way in which to calm his fears, discipline his mind and find release from the nightmares into which he has plunged. For me, Teilhard de Chardin has come closest to explaining the meaning of life and our relation to it. Some of his writings are difficult to interpret, as there is a mystical quality in them and he uses new words which are hard to understand. De Chardin was a mixture of scientist and priest and therefore more able to heal the rift between the two. He was a paleontologist with an international reputation but it was his philosophical and theological writings which had marked him out as one of the great thinkers of the twentieth century. His scientific background helped and did not hinder his concept of God.

With these thoughts in my mind I went back to the hospital after a meal to see how my operation cases were doing. Carrying a torch I made my way round the wards with Mark, stepping over recumbent forms, gently pulling back the blankets and enquiring of the nurse some details concerning pulse, temperature, haemorrhage and other vital facts which I needed to know. Most African patients pull up a blanket or sheet over their heads and seem to sleep like the dead. Considerable stimulation has to be applied if you are to discover how they are and what complaints they have. I fiddled with an intravenous drip by moving the needle in the vein. I was relieved to see it dripping again. Any operation tends to deplete the body of some fluid and it is important that it should be replaced as soon as possible in the post-operative period. If the patient can't or won't drink then his veins must be fed instead. Somalis particularly are very loathe to drink much by mouth. In such a hot climate this is strange but perhaps they know best how to deal with the heat of the desert.

Mark and I completed our rounds and then together recrossed the street to his house and mounted the long stone staircase to the roof. Everyone else was already on their camp beds in rows and thankfully I joined them. I lay back and lost my thoughts in the great canopy of stars overhead.

8
Safari Rally

My leisure moments were normally spent in the open, on the farm or reading in the peace of Ol Molog and I never thought that I should be involved in motor-car rallies, but when Robin became interested I got caught up in his enthusiasm and accompanied him from time to time as second driver or navigator, and helped him to get started in the sport. Robin, with his great mechanical ingenuity and quick reflexes, was a born racing driver. He understood cars instinctively and after the initial shock of being driven really fast, I too became used to it and had complete faith in his abilities. As a surgeon I had become horrified by the amount of time I had spent dealing with the end result of motor-car accidents and I had spent some time analysing the cause of accidents and discussing what could be done to cut down the appalling mortality on the roads. I learnt through the sport of rally driving that in most cases accidents are not caused by these good drivers. They are caused by people who have drunk too much or are on drugs or who have allowed their cars to become mechanically unsound and, of course, for many other reasons. Rally drivers are usually very fit, look after their cars because they are enthusiasts and, in fact, by and large, have a remarkably accident-free record. I did not believe this until I got involved in the sport but the statistics do show a very clean slate.

In East Africa, once a year, there is an international rally called the Safari Rally which has the reputation of being the toughest in the world. It has become the most popular sporting event of the year and in the end, through television and films, it is seen by four hundred million people around the world. The event started as the Coronation Safari Rally back in 1952 and was then a very different event from what it has become today. It started as a local rally over the Easter weekend and consisted of a couple of friends finding a car they were keen on and competing with other drivers around the amazing roads of East Africa. It was amateurish, great fun and a challenge to local talent. Everybody enjoyed it and nobody took it too seriously. At Easter time there is usually heavy rain and the earth roads of East Africa become like chocolate mousse of a particularly sticky kind. There is a great variety of different types of road surface and the altitude changes from sea level to 9000 feet in the Highlands so at one moment the temperature may be 100°F. and shortly afterwards you are up again in the mountains where the temperature may have dropped 60° or 70°. It was these amazing changes of dry and wet, hot and cold, plains and mountains, dust and mud intermingled together over five thousand kilometres which gave the Safari its unique appeal.

Gradually the event began to create greater interest and much of the credit must go to Eric Cecil, who became known as 'Mr Safari'. Eric, a Nairobi businessman, won the event himself in the early days, and gradually built up the Safari into the international rally it is today. It was a success story and he was helped by a growing band of enthusiasts. Perhaps many East Africans look back on the early days of the event with nostalgia and feel that its present atmosphere is too cut-throat, too commercial, and too expensive. This seems to be the inevitable course in international sport and if it is to remain on the international calendar it has to be this way – take it or leave it.

I came to the sport rather late and many people said to me, 'There's no fool like the old fool.' My family bore with me bravely and Robin was most considerate to his somewhat ancient father-in-law. We entered the 1968 Safari together when I was in my fiftieth year, but we had driven together the year before and had been pleased to finish a gruelling dry Safari in a small Peugeot 204. We won the prize for the highest-placed new entry to the Safari and got the much-coveted 'Finishers' badge.

Although the Safari is run at Easter time, preparations have to start early in the year. Perhaps it was this element of the sport which the family enjoyed most, the mounting excitement as their 'horse' came up to the starting line. The route is usually published some time in January, which gives competitors the chance to recce all the roads and make their own notes with the help of the official route notes. I enjoyed working on the details at the weekends, which meant getting out the maps, working out our refuelling stops, where we were going to meet our service cars, what spares we were going to carry, and a hundred and one other details. Careful planning is vital if you are to have any chance in finishing this marathon event. Robin and I were private entries, which meant getting our own car and meeting all the expenses ourselves. Even in those days it was an expensive affair; now it is almost prohibitive. The families, both Robin's and mine, were untiring in their efforts to see that we had everything we needed and without them we should not have got far.

In 1968 we did our recce in a number of different cars and only got the car in which we finally competed ten days before the start. These recces were all-important and had to be done at weekends when we could get off from work. I remember wandering around the Usambaras, the mountains west of Tanga, one night in the fog, after having completed a terrific mileage. We had become very sleepy and were wending our way back to the farm in the early hours of the morning. I noticed that Robin was beginning to feel the strain and I was having more and more difficulty in finding the route. Occasionally he would swerve for no apparent reason but I said nothing as any comment at this hour might have been misconstrued. Later Robin admitted that he had begun to see bears in the road but he would not admit this as he knew I would laugh at him, since bears do not frequent the continent of Africa. It turned out that he was having hallucinations from tiredness, but it did explain the mysterious bouts of swerving.

Our preparations went on apace as the day of the start drew near. Ten days before we were due to start we took delivery in Dar-es-Salaam of a Ford Cortina GT. Robin drove it back home and proceeded to tear it to pieces in the farm workshop. I cannot remember all that he did to our steed but he transformed it from a humdrum hack into a magnificent racehorse. It was a phenomenal transformation. All the weak places were spot-welded, tougher suspension was substituted, special lights were added, rally seats were put in, and in ten brief days Robin had done a prodigious task and had prepared a car which perhaps could last the course. We had had a final briefing meeting with all our friends who gave so much to see us through. Everyone knew what was expected of them, where they had to be at what time, whether we wanted coffee or Lucozade, how much fuel was required at such and such a place and when the servicing should be done and where.

The old hands in the Safari will always say, 'You have to finish if you are going to win.' This really means that you have to nurse your car, hold on and let your competitors destroy their cars by going too fast in the early stages. You have to play the waiting game but stay within striking distance all the time. For many years, the overseas professionals tended to overdo it at the start and go all out before they had given themselves a proper chance, while the local drivers who knew the conditions better held back until the field had thinned out and they could work out a strategy that would see them home. Perhaps nowadays this attitude is changing and the top drivers feel they have to go all out all the time if they are to stand a chance of winning. They rely on their servicing teams to rebuild the car if something fundamental goes wrong. Certainly the overseas drivers are doing much better now and on three occasions have won the event.

The great day finally came and the excitement rose to fever pitch. There were ninety-two cars entered and every indication that it was going to be a wet safari. The route took us out of Nairobi up to Limuru and the Kinangop through the Rift Valley up to Mau Narok and on through the Highlands, up the Nandi escarpment and on through into Uganda to Kampala where the first stop would occur. Then back round the country roads, across the slopes of Mount Elgon, skirting Kitale, down into the desert country through the Marech pass, up Chesangoch to Iten and then back down into the Kerio Valley again and up to Kabarnet and on eventually to Nakuru where there was another stop. Then on again up to Thompson's Falls, Nanyuki, round Mount Kenya along the treacherous windy road from Meru to Embu and finally back into Nairobi for our half-way rest.

It is masochistic sport and yet it has a great appeal. Perhaps the battling with the elements is part of the fun, but it is in essence an endurance test for man and his machine. From the spectators' points of view it clearly has enormous excitement, particularly if they know some of the competitors. For a whole weekend they dream they are behind the wheel of a safari car.

Waiting for the start is always the most trying time; nerves are taut and stretched and one's mind is obsessed with trying not to forget some essential item of equipment. At last we were off, car number 18, and we settled down to the first few miles of this gruelling event.

I remember that one front shock-absorber went early in the rally on the first evening after we had done less than a hundred miles. This was a bitter blow and eventually it had to be replaced. It delayed us, of course, but otherwise all was going well. Cars began to fall out for one reason or another, mechanical troubles being the most common at this stage. The roads were in a terrible state and the rain was intermittent, but hard at times. We had started at about 5.00 p.m. from the City Hall in Nairobi. The crowds had been terrific as we left the ramp and we knew how many people were listening in to the radio broadcasts and busily writing down the results and times on their score sheets. The public find this a particularly intriguing pastime as they record the favourites and compare the points lost by each car.

At Kampala, Robin and I were quite satisfied with our progress and we were determined to keep going as fast as we could but always nursing the car, because the rally had only just started and there was a long way to go.

The next leg through Uganda was very wet but Robin was a master in mud. He had learnt the technique from all the driving he had done on farm roads during the rains and seemed to be able to drive almost as fast in mud as in the dry. When the going gets very sticky there are a lot of techniques which help. Firstly, the car must have mud-grip tyres and a non-slip differential, and then it is essential to keep going and not spin the wheels which tends only to dig one deeper into the mire. These techniques are only learnt by experience. The rally cars are all fitted with steps on the back and straps to hang on by. The co-driver is expected to leap out and ride on the back of the car to keep the weight over the rear wheels which helps with the traction. It was an ungainly perch and became highly dangerous if the driver forgot that his companion was riding outside and accelerated after the muddy patch and started to drive at the usual frantic rally speeds.

The section in the Kerio Valley and up the Chesongoch pass was appalling. We lost a lot of time, but so did everyone else. The rocks in the road were hazardous, as were the places where the rivers crossed the route. During our recce we had been unable to get up the Chesongoch pass – the gear ratio had not been low enough, which gives an indication of its steepness. With a new bottom gear we got up this treacherous road, though to call it a road is a great compliment. It was more like an open drain. On one side there was a precipice and on the other a rock wall. In many areas it was impossible to consider passing and single file was the order of the day. This road has now been completely abandoned and washed away. It was one of the fiercest trials of the whole Safari. Up at the top the road was very slippery from rain but we got along steadily and then went back down into the Kerio Valley through Tambach and up to Kabarnet. A long stretch followed along the top of the ridge to Kipkorian. There was hardly more than one hundred yards of straight road – round and round the hairpins we went in a sort of mechanical trance. I was beginning to become totally disorientated. I found that one of the tasks of the navigator which I disliked most was switching my eyes from the road and back to my notes, especially at night. Robin and I had a system where I would call out the turn, T junction or crossroads in tenths of a mile from the globemaster. I would say three-tenths to a sharp left turn then two-tenths and then one-tenth and Robin would know when to start braking. It was a responsible job and absolute concentration was required to avoid causing an accident by calling the wrong distance or the wrong turn. I cannot remember this nightmare section very well but I do remember vividly the feeling of relief when Nakuru finally came into sight. Food and drink were the first necessity and to sit still for a brief period was a welcome relief. We were full of questions to our friends and supporters.

'How is No. 7 doing?'

'Are we ahead of No. 21?'

When you are actually in the rally, it is very difficult to reckon how you are going in relation to other cars, but the spectators know the position much better than the competitors. I finally got into a bath and went straight to sleep and had to be woken by Robin in order to get to the car in time for the hazardous run round Mount Kenya.

The second night always seems to be worst and it needs great willpower to force yourself to stay awake. I remember seeing a powerful light some way off pointing straight down the road. We were doing about 100 m.p.h. and only at the last moment did Robin realize that in fact the light was on a tractor ploughing in a field and that the road actually bore sharply to the right. How he got the car round that corner I shall never know. On we sped and my most lasting memory concerns that awful road from Meru to Embu which has ninety-nine hairpin bends. It had rained buckets and the surface was glass-like. In order to stay on the road at all we let the pressure in the tyres right down to ten pounds. It was a nightmare and the death-knell of numerous cars. We helped pull out a number of our friends and finally got through, though we lost an hour and twenty minutes on the section. When we arrived in Nairobi we found that there were only twenty cars left to start on the second half of the rally eight hours later and many of these were in poor shape. A quick sleeping pill and then oblivion. Robin had managed to keep our Ford in very good order and at least we were starting on the second half with a chance of finishing. Little did we realize that the heavens were going to open and at one point ten inches of rain would fall in the night and wash away everything, including a large section of tarmac road.

I always remember a poor retired rally driver who was hauled to the radio studio to give the public his view of the rally. He may have lost everything else but he retained his sense of humour. 'Mr X,' said the interviewer, 'what did you think of the route?' and Mr X replied, 'Well – when I found my sandwiches floating around under my armpits in the car, I realized there was no future to motoring.'

This sounds like an exaggeration but on two occasions we had water right over the bonnet. I foolishly opened the door on one of these occasions to get out and push and all my notes started floating around in the water with my maps.

Drivers tend to become somewhat laconic when they are interviewed by the press at a time when they are dead beat and heading for their beds or a cup of coffee. I overheard a friend of mine after the rally was over and we had been swimming in floods for forty-eight hours, being questioned by a reporter who said, 'Was it wet on the southern leg?'

'No, no,' said my friend, 'only a very heavy dew.' This was assiduously written down and the reporter went off happy with his tit-bit.

We started off again on Saturday night and soon we passed two more cars, one of which belonged to the overseas favourite. There were, now, no overseas competitors left. We struggled across the black cotton soil to Loitokitok on Kilimanjaro and down to Himo and then back towards the coast. The roads were no longer roads but river beds. We went round through Rukanga and I felt sure we were about to get permanently stuck. With consummate skill Robin got us back on to the main Mombasa road. It was a real relief to have a few miles of tarmac.

On we drove through the night, the third night now of this endurance test, and back into Tanzania on the coast road and finally to the bottom of the famous Usambara Mountains on the east side. We knew we were in for major trouble here and sure enough it came. There was a flat plain which had flooded and there was the black cotton soil to deal with again. By this time the Safari was down to ten cars. Most cars were pulled through this section by a tractor and I believe Robin was the only driver to negotiate it under his own steam.

Then we climbed a very steep escarpment ten miles in length. The surface was appalling. The Ford was low geared and we slipped past three of our competitors, but pride came before the fall for when we reached the top, we were boiling. We stopped and filled up with water – one of the hoses was leaking. Robin fixed it and on we went through the slush and mud. The Usambaras were non-stop torture. Fog, rain, pot holes, punctures – we had the lot. I do not remember how I found the way through these tea estates – they were awash. There were wash-aways, rock falls and every type of hazard. If we had been a few hours later it would have been impassable as this was the area in which the ten inches of rain fell that night.

Somehow we reached Korogwe and were met by the family who plied us with hot drinks, and washed the lights and windscreen. We were totally exhausted. Robin's face was white, his eyes red and strained, and a fiercesome growth of beard had appeared to make him look a real desperado.

The car was serviced by the Ford service crew. What luxury – at last we were getting some professional help. A face came in through the window and said, 'Mike, you are terrific – sit where you are and if necessary we'll carry the car to the finish.'

What cheer this was. We had allies who were determined to get our car home. It gave us new heart and we staggered on down to Dar-es-Salaam. Our car now had new wheels and tyres, had been thoroughly checked and everything was going well.

After a brief rest, we turned home for the final seven hundred miles or so to Nairobi. We started off to the west and before long got hopelessly stuck in a sisal estate. The ruts were so deep that the car bellied and no further progress was possible. We had to get out and jack the back of the car till it was above the ruts and then push it sideways off the jack so that the wheels came down on the higher ground between the ruts. Then we went round the front and did the same thing there. I cannot remember how many times we did this manœuvre but finally the road gave out completely. It was my worst moment. I had got us lost – oh! what awful agony and despair. I started to apologize and could barely look Robin in the face.

'Hold on,' he said, 'I am going to have a look around; give me the torch.' I stayed by the car, sick with humiliation; we were over three-quarters of the way round the course and I had lost the route. It was dark, raining and generally miserable. Suddenly I heard a shout from Robin but I could not hear what he said. He came splashing back. 'I've found the tyre marks,' he said. 'There's been a wash-away.'

My spirits rose as I sensed that salvation might be at hand. We set off together and had another look. There was a four-foot drop in the road and twenty yards farther on the road started again and there were the tyre marks. Robin said, 'Look, Mike, our only hope is to go back a bit and take a run at it and see if we can jump the ditch here.'

This sounded suicide to me but I was too far gone to mind, even really to register. We backed for about two hundred yards and then Robin got into first gear, revved up the engine and off we went – into second gear and then at about 40 m.p.h. we took to the air. We were over – we came down with a crunch but the suspension held and we were off again. Shortly afterwards I recognized a turning I knew and I realized we were still on the route. Not long after this we came across some of our fellow competitors beside their cars with a gloomy look on their faces. Apparently one car was axle deep in mud and unable to get out and everyone else was queued up behind him. There was no way round as there was a river on one side and a bank on the other. This looked like the end for us all. We were at the bottom of a steep rise and each car would need a run at it. As always in Africa people started appearing out of the bush. In the end we had fifty splendid men and we lifted the stuck car bodily from its grave. There was hope still. We got him up the hill and we all managed to follow but finally all hope disappeared as we sank into impossible ruts. A lorry must have gone along this road, known as the Kiroka Pass, earlier on, and dug ruts which we could not cope with. Just as we really felt that we might as well go to sleep in our cars and wait for the dawn, a tractor arrived. It had been sent back down the road by the organizers when they realized that the remaining competitors were finally bogged down for good.

One by one we were pulled through the mire until we came to a place where we could start again and get moving under our own steam. By this time our car was beginning to feel the appalling punishment we had given it. Our front off-side wheel was well out of alignment – something was badly bent. She became a beast to drive and we went through tyres at a great rate.

Through Morogoro and on up to Handeni and finally back to Korogwe at dawn – could we last the course? It looked very doubtful – the car was giving increasing trouble and small wonder, after driving up and down river beds for hundreds of miles.

Three hundred miles to go and nothing really difficult in the way of roads. We were determined to finish. We were serviced in Korogwe and had something to drink. The family again were magnificent – they had had a terrible time too, waiting in the rain for us and exhausted with their efforts to cut us off and be in time to meet us. Tempers were beginning to fray, especially as the enormous crowds gave us no room to manœuvre.

A few miles out of Korogwe we saw a sight which convinced me that we were having hallucinations. I rubbed my eyes – could that be an African hut coming across the road? No, impossible, and yet there was another. We stopped, got out and walked to a place where the tarmac ended abruptly. Looking ahead about three hundred yards I could see the tarmac start again but in between there was a rushing roaring brown torrent which we gauged was about five feet deep. Again we faced the fact that we would be time-barred and have to retire. We were speechless with disappointment. We sat in the car and tried to be philosophical. It was no good. We were tired, angry, filthy and totally thwarted by this last turn of the fates.

All we could do was to wait for the torrent to subside. We realized that this was the end result of the ten-inch rainfall in the hills above. After two hours' wait I climbed down into the torrent and started wading across the gap. Was it possible for a car to follow? I thought not. Robin thought otherwise and I watched with horror as he slowly let the car down over the edge and started into the torrent. I tried to find the smoothest way through the water – I slipped and got soaked but on Robin came. I could scarcely believe that any car could do this. Water was building up on the upper side – would the car simply be washed away and down into the main river below? No, he was through and up the bank on the far side. The car stood on dry ground. We walked round it and Robin got underneath. It would still go but we could make no speed. We limped on and after a bit it seemed to be going better again. Eventually we arrived back in our own home country around Kilimanjaro and had a great reception at 'Dutch Corner' where the road took off westwards towards Mount Meru. Robin knew every corner of this country as he had been born not far away. We began to make good progress again. Up over Momella and down to Arusha we went. A car went out at Usa River with a con rod through the side of the engine. We were down to seven. It was like the song of the ten little nigger boys.

In Arusha we had to have some fundamental things done to the car if we were to get back to Nairobi. We were one and a half hours in the garage. Everyone was frantic with exhaustion but we were so nearly home, we must finish.

At last we were on the road again – the final blow hit us, both rear shock-absorbers came through the boot. We could only drive at 40 m.p.h. because above that speed the car became uncontrollable. Back into Kenya at Namonga and up the earth road to Kajiado we toiled. I looked at Robin and I saw through all his tiredness a new light in his expression. We were going to make it.

Then the crowds began to grow and soon we were totally submerged by thousands of onlookers. We sounded the horn, we banged on the roof – please give us some room. For fifteen miles we drove like this and then at last there was the ramp outside the Nairobi City Hall and we were sitting on the roof of the car sipping champagne. The crowd was mad with excitement. For three days and four nights they had followed this epic Safari on their radios and by the roadside. The family were there, bruised, battered, but tremendously happy that we had come through against all odds.

And so the legend of the 'Unsinkable Seven' was born. We had been part of it and as we were carried off at last to bed, the horror of that drive was forgotten and only the pleasure of survival remained.

9
Raising the Wind

As I sat in the Swissair D.10 flying towards Europe at the beginning of a new fund-raising trip, I shut my eyes and relived this last day in Africa because I knew that my immediate task was to try and bring this picture with me and make it live in the minds of the many supporters of our medical work in North America and Europe. I had to try and find inspiration somewhere, though all I felt at that moment was fatigue. Before leaving Africa there are always a host of jobs to be finished and instructions to be left and I still felt bemused in my mind. I must now re-orientate and make the jump between the two cultures, the two ways of living and the two ways of thinking.

As I began to relax in my seat and as the aircraft levelled out at the top of its climb, the various activities and projects of the Foundation began to appear before me and I seized on them to try and mould them into some shape which would be recognizable in the places which I was about to visit.

What had happened during the last fourteen hours? Did it fall into a recognizable cohesive plan? It did, but only if you could view the whole canvas and paint in the various scenes as part of the larger picture.

I thought first of the training and the seminars which were going on in our training centre in Nairobi. Groups of doctors and administrators were coming in for courses on medical administration. They came from each province. In medical school you never learn anything about administration or medical economics, and yet, certainly in developing countries, you are immersed in these subjects directly you take up the position of a district medical officer. You have to learn to live within a budget, organize your staff and deal with all their problems. You have to work out a routine and keep it, run an orderly office and know what is going on in each department which has a bearing on your work.

Looking down I saw Lake Turkana off our starboard wing and for a time my concentration wavered but the scene below helped me realize once again that communications were a vital aspect of our work and essential if we were to overcome some of the obstacles which lay below in this vast arid stretch of country.

Immediately this brought to mind our Flying Doctor Service with its aircraft and radio network and a staff which now knew the country intimately. We had been fortunate in developing a team of young pilots who had been brought up in East Africa, spoke Swahili, and by dint of experience had learnt the art of the bush pilot while at the same time passing all their senior licences which would enable them to fly with the airlines when they chose to. Nurses ran the radio room because we learnt that it was necessary to have people who could interpret the medical messages coming over the radio. They did it well and managed to convey to the seventy-four stations which used our network that they were there to help. This meant patience, tact and local knowledge. I remembered that earlier that day I had been called to the radio to discuss a patient with a doctor at a mission hospital. I had sat down in front of the radio and said, 'Maua, this is Michael Wood, go ahead with your message, over.'

'Good morning, Mr Wood,' came back the doctor's voice. 'Sorry to bother you with this problem. We have a man with head injuries and we are not sure whether to ask you to evacuate him to Nairobi or whether we should look after him here and save him a trip by air, over.'

'Please tell me his history, signs and symptoms, over.'

'He was injured yesterday and has been partially unconscious since. He is restless and has a depressed fracture on X-ray over the left parietal region, over.'

'Has he any signs of compression? Over.'

'Not really, his pupils are equal and react to light, and his pulse is normal, over.'

'Have you got the instruments for elevating the fracture? Over.'

'Some of them. What do we need? Over.'

'You should have a drill and some burrs . . .' I went on to describe the technique of the operation.

'What do we do if we find there is haemorrhage? Over,' came the doctor's voice.

'Wash out the clot with warm saline solution and see if you can discover where the bleeding is coming from.' Finally the doctor agreed to undertake the operation and made a great success of it and the patient recovered.

Other similar conversations occupied my attention for a time and I felt immensely grateful for that radio network which had been such a lifeline on countless occasions.

The aircraft of the Flying Doctor Service had been busy during the day, though there had been one snag with one of the Cessna 402s which had necessitated putting the aircraft up on jacks and replacing an essential part which had become worn in the undercarriage. This had taken all day, as the spare part was not easily available and had taken some time to locate.

One aircraft was with a surgical team in central Tanzania. I had seen the operating list which looked formidable and would take at least two days to complete. There had been two emergencies which occupied two other aircraft. One had to go to Kisii to pick up a child with polio. This mission had been successfully accomplished and the child was in Nairobi in a respirator. The other emergency involved a car accident on the Mombasa road. Too often we were called to deal with these accidents but in this case a young African woman had sustained a fractured vertebra. She, too, was back now in hospital under treatment.

Yet another aircraft had taken a reconstructive surgeon to a hospital in the bush to work on leprosy problems, operating, teaching, checking the physiotherapy techniques and encouraging the patients to show initiative and help themselves.

As I recalled these sorties from the comfort of my seat above the clouds, the realization came to me that the Flying Doctor Service had now become an integral part of the medical life of East Africa. It was needed and it was doing a unique job.

I knew that the Medical Director had, during the day, been carrying on important negotiations concerning our big new project at Kibwezi, an area half-way between Nairobi and the coast where we had been asked to run a comprehensive health service for a population of one hundred thousand people living in this arid, unproductive area. He would be discussing today the question of staff housing for the health centre we were planning to build. It had to fit into the Government pattern and we wanted to find out how much it was going to cost us.

As my flight continued over the Sudan, I sensed a great feeling of relief because I knew that the administration team in Nairobi really had a grip on our whole operation and that our finances were in good safe hands. Previously, when I had had to do these jobs myself but less well, I never felt happy about leaving for too long. It was a sign of the growing maturity of our whole operation. I had, at last, got the right people in the right jobs.

Where was the Maasai mobile unit? I tried to think when they had set out again on their monthly safari. Again, I knew with confidence that this team, which had been working together for over ten years, were fully prepared for every contingency. They would be welcome wherever they went because they were known and respected all over Maasailand. They knew the people and the roads and what they were likely to have to do. This compact, well-equipped unit had learnt by dint of experience how to deal with their nomadic patients and how to look after themselves in the bush. They had coped with lions, with floods, with famine and with epidemics. I thought to myself that I must go down and visit them when I got back from my fund-raising trip. In previous times whenever I had been able to go and see them, I had always learnt a lot myself, particularly in the art of handling people. Yes, they were a team of which we were all immensely proud.

I thought too, as my plane flew smoothly on to the north, of our Somali team working out in Garissa in another mobile unit. They had the great problem of tuberculosis to deal with, finding new cases, following up old ones to see they had their medicines, checking on the sputum to see if the TB bacillus was present. This was a tough job in hot, dusty, unrelenting country. Our team was entirely African and a further proof that our Africanization programme was justified.

Our health education team would be in Kakamega helping to educate a group of mothers there. Of all our projects, in the long run perhaps this was the most important. It would not be dramatic but it would slowly be getting at the root of the health problem. Africans teaching Africans about nutrition, family planning, water supplies and all the other basic health needs of a developing country.

I knew too that there was a flight clinic down at Shombole just north of Lake Natron. We had made a strip there and were getting access to a large group of people who had no medical help. One day, when there were sufficient static services, our mobile approach could be dispensed with, but not yet.

I was beginning to get sleepy but my mind would still not let me rest. A picture of the workers in the Flying Doctor Society packing up Christmas cards flashed through my mind. This society had proved a great success, raising over £20,000 a year to help with the running expenses of the service. The Christmas cards, designed especially by local artists, had been well received by the public and close on one hundred thousand would be sold in the next few weeks. I felt so grateful to Maddie de Mott for the generous way she continues to give her time freely to this enterprise.

Then I thought of those last few hours in the office with my secretary and the information officer, both invaluable people in the team. A secretary, who becomes a personal assistant, acts as your right hand. She saves much time and smooths the way through the day. If she can think for you, as mine does, she can prevent you from making awful errors, she can protect you from unnecessary time-consuming chores and be the height of tact when you are late or in the wrong place. I realized, as I slowly sank into sleep, that I owed my secretary so much for keeping me relatively sane. At the last moment there was my ticket, my passport, my health documents and list of addresses. The files I needed had been stacked on my desk and the information officer had brought me all the various documents I needed to take to the overseas offices which I was about to visit. Photographs. newsletters, annual reports, manuals and all the other paraphernalia essential to my fund-raising job.

'Are the budget papers in?' I had asked.

'Yes, they are in the files,' came the confident reply.

'Mr Wood, you said you had to speak to the Iranian Ambassador before you left,' prompted my secretary. The last telephone call had been made and there I was, at last, fully equipped as a travelling salesman.

My staff looked at me, I suspected, in a rather pitying fashion as we had said goodbye. I think they wondered how I could possibly manage without them. They were, of course, right. I could not manage without them but I knew that now I was going to be passed on through the AMREF network overseas and they were all used to dealing with the peripatetic director-general whose foibles and inefficiencies were well known to them. I was in good hands and so thankful that at last an international team of helpers had been built up who could do so much of the preparatory work for me.

With these final fleeting thoughts, I fell asleep. I am lucky in being able to sleep in jets and I do not suffer unduly from the so-called jet-lag. I did not even dream, and my next conscious moment was being woken by the air hostess who asked me to fasten my seat belt as we were about to land at Zurich. I got out and breathed the Alpine air and allowed the metamorphosis to take place. I had to be like a chameleon and take on the local colour. I must now condition myself to interpreting what was going on in Africa to all the people I would be seeing. It would be different in every country, because each country had a different approach to fund-raising. I had to try and enthuse them with my enthusiasm and relate to them what had passed through my mind on my way from Africa. The background would need to be sketched in and photographs, slides and films would help in this task. I would have to describe in detail the projects in which they were interested and report on how much progress had been made and what was happening to the funds.

Although I had done this many times before, I was always diffident about my ability to put it across. This diffidence would shrink as I got into my stride. I found I was most articulate when I was speaking to small interested groups. The physical proximity of my audience always had an effect. If I could lean across a table and speak to a board of directors I was happier, but if I had to speak in a cold hall without being able to get the atmosphere or the mood of my audience, I found I got more and more lost and unable to conjure up the magic of Africa and make anyone excited about it.

In Switzerland I was going for meetings at the World Health Organization in Geneva. There was no difficulty here as they knew the problems and we talked the same language. I was also going to see a great helper of ours in Bern who had seen the work and was an enthusiastic supporter. In fact, to use a cricketing term, the first over was going to be straightforward.

Then I would be in Munich where again I would be among friends who knew me and the work. The approach would be different, especially with the Government, who sometimes gave the impression that they thought we were boy scouts and really the whole thing would be better if it was done on a government-to-government basis. They were interested in the whole problem of 'infrastructure' and their help tended to go to training and social work. Also at the back of their minds would be the thought that this is an English organization and we would have to convince them that in fact it was an international agency with a strong German contingent. There would be the old question about aeroplanes and how expensive they were and I would trot out the figures to show that we could fly as cheaply as we could drive on the roads, with the added advantage of saving the doctor's time. The Church organizations had been most helpful and understanding and appreciated what had been done by AMREF with the missions. Here I would find I was talking to professionals who knew the conditions under which we worked and had visited the field operations in Africa. We might have differences of opinion on priorities but there would not be any major problems.

Then there was the new idea of trying to get an organization started in Austria. This would be covering new ground, although the Austrian Ambassador had given me encouragement to try.

America would be entirely different for many reasons. It was such a big country that it was difficult to know where to start. America had had a different historical role from Europe in its relations with Africa and again fund-raising was more professional and competitive than anywhere else. The Board of Directors of the Foundation in America had had an uphill struggle to interest Americans in our work in Africa. They had stuck to it in a most commendable fashion and recently their efforts were being increasingly rewarded. I would be given a tight schedule, very good briefing and a number of people to come with me to tackle the Foundations which were our main supporters. Within two weeks they would ask me to go and see a dozen Foundations where appointments had been arranged. Within this time I would be going to Detroit, Pittsburgh, Dayton and Washington and, of course, having planning meetings with my friends and helpers.

Canada would be different again. There are fewer Foundations to approach but Canada, through the Commonwealth connection, has played an increasing role in foreign aid to Africa. The Kiwanis Clubs had been staunch supporters and the 'Miles for Millions' walk in Toronto had produced a useful income for us each year. The Canadian International Development Agency had begun to show interest in our programme and helped to fund two projects. But more importantly the Board of Directors there had a growing expertise and their chairman was a dedicated man who had a very wide experience of voluntary work around the world. I believe that we were poised to expand our appeal in Canada but that much preparation would be needed first.

And then back to Europe to our annual international meeting in Copenhagen. It would be like a large family get-together. We would learn from each other and discuss the future policy and its financial implications. It was fitting that Denmark should be the country in which we would meet, as this small country had given us the largest grant which had enabled us to do so many new things. In particular they had built the Training Centre, hostel and offices. I was determined to give a good account of how we had used this generous gift. Our committee in Denmark was relatively new and already they had set themselves a target for raising an endowment fund to help the medical work in Africa. I knew, too, that the meeting would be well arranged because I had heard about some of the preparations. Perhaps we would discover new methods of co-operation and certainly much would be achieved outside the formal meetings as well as inside.

It seemed, too, that interest was growing in Sweden. The Swedes have done such a remarkable work in Eastern Africa which they had chosen as one part of the world on which to concentrate their aid. It was clear that the countries which had no colonial past were more acceptable in many parts of Africa and this was particularly true of Scandinavia.

I had planned, too, to go and see old friends in Norway and visit the Norwegian Church Relief Organization. The Lutheran Church in Scandinavia had always been great supporters and we had enjoyed being able to assist them in their mission hospitals in Africa. I had a soft spot for Haydom, the Norwegian Lutheran Hospital in the Mbulu District in Tanzania. I had seen it grow and flourish in a most remote area. The extensions to the hospital had been opened by President Julius Nyerere. Before his visit four bulldozers had arrived to improve the mission airstrip so that the President could land in safety. I remembered shaking the President by the hand on that day and suggesting that he visited some other mission hospitals so that we would get the airstrips done up there as well. He laughed and said he would do his best.

Then back to England in time to hear Alfred Brendel play a concert for us in the Civic Hall at Guildford. This generous gesture was going to help the English office with their fund-raising. Having spent some ten years in London as a medical student and trainee surgeon, it was, of course, like going home. The English end had been founded by my old teacher and friend, Archie McIndoe, who had gathered around him a number of friends and begun to work out of the Royal College of Surgeons in the late fifties. It had come a long way since then and had been supported by a growing number of people and organizations. We had just received a splendid gift of an Islander aircraft from the British Government which had been a great encouragement to us in Africa. We were fortunate, too, in having two full-time staff members in London who, with an active Board, had begun to raise an increasing amount of funds despite the depressed condition of the British economy. It must be remembered that Britain had had a closer relationship with East Africa than any other of the countries which supported us, and that therefore there was a built-in interest, as so many British people had lived in East Africa or had business interests there.

On my way home to Africa I would be spending a week in Abu Dhabi in the Gulf to start work on a survey to advise the Government on the possibilities of a mobile health service. I also hoped to interest the Government in financing our project at Kibwezi.

As I prepared to embark on this fund-raising trip, I had high hopes because I had witnessed the growth and increasing interest which was being shown around the world in our small efforts and I sensed that the developed world realized more and more their commitment to the third world. I knew that the interest was not entirely philanthropic and that there was a large element of enlightened self-interest. After all, who was the developed world going to trade with if the third world went under and became a bankrupt and famine-stricken zone? The Lomé convention gave me hope that Europe now realized that a much bigger programme was required to help Africa, just as the USA had realized that Marshall Aid was the way to help Europe back on its feet after the Second World War. Certainly it was generous but it was also in the best interests of America. Interdependence between countries and continents is slowly becoming a recognized reality, despite the stresses and strains which are very evident in many parts of the world and threaten to tear us all apart.

I had been fortunate in being allowed to see some of the schemes in which I had taken part flourish and grow. No one could ever take away the enormous pleasure and interest in developing ten thousand acres on Kilimanjaro or working out the beginning of a medical Foundation in Africa or flying around the continent and lending a hand with development schemes here and there or educating four children and seeing them take their place in the world. With these thoughts in my mind I felt both humble and grateful and ready to take the next step.

In the early days, and even up to today, I have found myself constantly torn in two by the need to help with the job in Africa and at the same time raise the money overseas to keep that job going. It has led to a permanent state of schizophrenia which I have never been able to resolve. While in Africa and seeing the overdraft grow, I have felt compelled to rush off to my good friends around the world and ask for their financial assistance, but when I get there I immediately feel the need to return to Africa to my post which I have deserted. It is so much easier to do the job than talk about it. No one in their senses likes soliciting for funds, yet what voluntary agency can survive without them? The one compensating feature has been the opportunity to meet a wonderful selection of people without whose help the Foundation would have been sunk without trace. It is because of my great respect for their selfless work that I attempt to write about the way this network emerged. 'The healing of the world is in its nameless saints.' Almost unconsciously people of many different backgrounds realize that they need to sacrifice something in order to preserve that essence which makes life worth living. It is indefinable but very real. The welfare state does not answer all the problems of existence; we feel the need to do something towards our salvation.

When I began to explain in a halting fashion what AMREF was trying to do, sometimes the spark caught and the recognition of the problem was immediate and spontaneous. This is always an exciting moment in human affairs as another kindred spirit is inspanned. I was constantly amazed at the interest which was engendered though of course often I was turned down flat. I began to grow a thicker skin as I realized that I must expect to be turned down nine times out of ten. It always used to amuse me how difficult people find it is to say 'No.' There are many ways of saying it and I think I now must know them all.

'Dr Wood,' a Foundation executive would say to me in New York, 'we think your scheme is a very attractive one but unfortunately we have spent all our available funds for this year. Do come and see us next year.' Or another executive would say, 'Dr Wood, what a pity you didn't come last month when we were deciding how to spend our grants for the next year.' Or even, 'Well, Dr Wood, your project doesn't really fit into our general policy but I know just the man you should see. I am sure he will help you. I will give you his name. He is Mr A working in the Z Foundation.'

On and on went the run around but I began to learn certain techniques. For instance, sometimes the Foundation executive who was given the job of seeing me would say, 'I find your project extremely interesting but unfortunately the policy of my board is not to give to medicine for the time being. If your project had concerned education perhaps . . .' Out of my pocket I would produce another project on education. My shoe leather began to wear thin as my skin got thicker. It was like playing a game of poker with the other chap holding all the aces. I had rather a penchant for poker. The secret is to fix your opponent with a guileless but gimlet-like gaze and use the art of bluff to a scandalous degree but always remember to produce the real cards when you can. The variations of this most subtle of games are infinite – so it is with donor agencies. Occasionally I got through to the funds, not often, but enough to keep things going at the African end. As our work output increased in Africa so the fund-raising became easier, as nothing succeeds like success. Sometimes at the end of a day trying to sell AMREF I became hoarse with repeating the same story. I always feared the question, 'Tell me, Dr Wood, what exactly does the AMREF do?' I could hear the click in my brain and the gramophone record would start all over again. 'Well, you see, we are engaged in taking medical care to the remote parts of East Africa . . .' I could hear my voice trailing on in a monotonous fashion as if I was reciting a boring poem and I became quite detached and could look down on myself as in a dream.

Perhaps the only times I really succeeded was with organizations who were so fed up with seeing me time and time again that they felt it was easier to pay me to go away. I went.

I felt sorry for these poor Foundation executives who were badgered by every good cause from all over the globe. They remained ever polite and gracious and did their level best to appear interested. I swore early on in this game that one day I would sit on the other side of the table. In this I have succeeded and when people come to me asking for support I have the answer ready on the tip of my tongue. 'Well, Dr C, I am very interested in your project but my board has allocated all our funds for this year. Perhaps if you called back next year, or I could recommend you going to see Mr D of the Y Foundation. I will give him a call and explain your project.'

Each country has its own technique and certain rules which you must obey if you are ever to hit the jackpot. Gradually my friends learned that I did have a story to tell and they rallied round to help. In fact they have done all the hard work and preparation which I have used to do some of the final soliciting. I learnt that it was very difficult to ask people to fund-raise for you unless you were prepared to go and give the authentic touch of the man who is doing the job. You can't fund-raise second-hand. Most donors want to talk to the people who actually do the work and are responsible for the projects. This is very natural and understandable but it means being prepared for a good mileage during the year.

As I travelled round the world begging for help wherever I could, I found myself also being able on the odd occasions to offer some suggestions on problems on which AMREF had developed some expertise.

The logistics involved in getting doctors, nurses and their equipment to where they are wanted at the right time can be more difficult than they sound. As a peripatetic doctor, it has fallen to my lot to discuss these issues in many parts of the world apart from our own back yard in Africa. AMREF has been asked to give advice to the medical authorities in places as far apart as the Ryukyu Islands in the Pacific, Iceland, Peru and Abu Dhabi. Although the local conditions in these places differ markedly, the problem to be overcome is much the same.

In the Pacific the problem concerned getting medical help to seventy-three islands on most of which no airstrip could be built. This meant helicopters and I had several fascinating days with my American friends there working out a scheme which finally went to the Cabinet. Two first-rate American helicopter pilots flew us around over the choppy blue sea and I began to learn some of the reasons why helicopters are not as safe as fixed-wing aircraft. For one thing, if the engine stops you can only glide twice the distance you are above the ground or sea at the time, while in aircraft this distance is about ten miles. Nevertheless, for the purpose we required them, nothing else would do. I worked out the distances, the cost and the radio network, and had many discussions with the health authorities and local doctors. I learnt that about three times in the year Okinawa was hit by tornadoes. Fortunately there was usually at least forty-eight hours' warning from the meteorological department. The winds were so strong that all the American Air Force and army planes were flown off the island to Taiwan because the risk of damage was so great. Apparently the tornado usually lasted about three days so you had to bring in provisions, tie everything down and sit it out in the houses until the winds subsided. It was impossible to walk on the streets without getting blown away. The tiles on the roofs were cemented on because otherwise they stood no chance. My visit did not coincide with one of these freaks of nature, for which I was thankful, but I did see the crops which had been flattened by the previous storms, especially the sugar. This must be a depressing feature for the island farmers.

In Iceland I was asked to give a lecture to the Icelandic Medical Association, which I did, and the following day I was flown round the island in a twin Comanche to see some of the problems which were involved with this difficult terrain. I learnt that for three months in the year there are terrifying blizzards which make all flying impossible. On the day that I visited the north coast of Iceland, I saw solid ice stretching out towards Greenland, and if you were foolhardy enough it was theoretically possible to walk all the way there. It had been a hard winter and the ice had come down unusually far south. My mind began to dwell on the problem of what you could do to help an isolated community of fifty souls if some accident should befall them in winter. Clearly there was no hope of getting there through the air even in a helicopter. Radio communication would help so that a doctor could advise what best to do. Each community needed to be well stocked with medical supplies and hopefully a nurse or someone with some medical knowledge would be living in the community. Women about to give birth should obviously be sent out before the winter closed in. These precautions seemed the only ones likely to be helpful.

As we flew over the central glaciers down to the south coast I couldn't help thinking of the Vikings who had rowed out from Scandinavia in open boats to find their future in the west. I had seen one of these famous boats in a museum in Oslo. What courage they must have possessed. What did they take with them? I suppose many of them were lost and never returned home – we shall never know. These were the men who set out to discover the coast of North America a thousand years ago. The famous sagas which have been handed down tell of these stirring times. The Icelandic terrain is barren and treeless but with a strange beauty of its own enhanced by the permanent glaciers and mountains which rise from the sea all round the island, particularly in the south. One feature which I remember well from this cursory glance was the rivers pouring off the glaciers all along the south coast and down into the sea. This brief visit has encouraged me to go again, spend more time and perhaps catch a salmon in those icy rivers.

In England some of the Foundations have been a great source of support, as have been other international agencies such as Oxfam. Oxfam is a household word in England as it has been a very successful agency raising over £6 million a year, but more important than this it has done an astounding job in educating the British public to an understanding of the predicament of the third world. There are, of course, others doing the same good work but none has been more successful than Oxfam. Over the years they have been constantly generous to AMREF and we have tried to keep faith with them by spending their money wisely and accounting for it accurately and promptly. There is no nonsense about Oxfam as they know their job, work hard at it, and are conspicuously careful about not wasting money on frills such as smart offices; and they help to guard the conscience of Britain in this difficult period in British history, as the retreat from the Empire is almost complete and yet much of the job once done by that Empire still needs to be done, albeit in a different way and under totally different conditions. You would not expect such an organization to escape all criticism. Doubtless mistakes have been made, but they are such a small element in the total force for good for which Oxfam stands. I have never quite understood the disgust and disdain with which people mention the term 'do-gooders'. Perhaps they are more in favour of the do-badders – after all there are plenty of them.

In each country where AMREF started a supporting committee steps were taken to set up and register a proper organization with recognized charitable status. All this took a little time and these eight organizations now meet once a year as the African Medical and Research Foundation International to discuss overall policy, debate the budget for the work in Africa and share out the responsibility of raising the necessary funds. Fortunately, over the last few years, the Governments of Kenya and Tanzania have also joined in to support the work. This has been an enormous encouragement to us, as it endorses the role we are playing and helps to give confidence to other countries who are considering helping us. The work done by this gallant band of supporters needs a book of its own but when I consider the time, energy and willing service they have given for so long I feel very humble. It is not possible to express adequately what is their due. I can only hope that the success of the venture is some reward.

Antoine de Saint-Exupery in one of his books said, 'The paradoxical truth seems to me of considerable psychological importance : that man's happiness lies not in freedom but in the acceptance of a duty.' This thought surely applies to all those who, in one way or another, have accepted the duty of helping humanity by giving of their time, energy and money to the many good causes which cry out for such help.

10
Sun, Storm and Fire

I often remember a story told by Saint-Exupery of his crash in the North African desert and how he and his navigator had to make a one-hundred-and-twenty-mile walk with no water. They had been lucky to escape but went through all the torments of hell from appalling thirst during the ensuing days. Their water bottles had burst in the crash and the water had seeped away into the sand so they had nothing left to drink except a half-bottle of wine. He describes how the tongue becomes like plaster of Paris, the saliva dries up, swallowing becomes impossible and finally a dry cough heralds the onset of death, which can only then be a blessed relief. With these gruesome thoughts travelling through my mind, I was determined always to check the water supply we carried on all our flights. It could make the whole difference to survival if ever a plane had to make a forced landing in the desert areas which we crossed nearly every day. I had once been to a lecture on survival given by an RAF officer and had learnt the various things which you can do which make survival more likely. Most of them are common sense, but panic tends to take over and people can do very stupid things unless they have been forced to study the problem. Nowadays we have small beacons in our planes which can be switched on and work off batteries. Any aircraft can pick up the 'bleep' noise and home in on the grounded plane. This is a great advance and the Flying Doctor

Service insists on fitting these gadgets to each of the planes. Perhaps the most useful tip is to realize that staying by the aeroplane is usually the wisest thing to do. There are exceptions but not many. Recently on two occasions I have noticed that planes have been found after having to come down in forest or desert but the occupants have been missing. If they had stayed by their plane they would have been rescued; as it was they died.

A message once came in from the police that there was a party missing somewhere at the south end of Lake Natron. It transpired that this party had been expected back by their friends three days previously; the friends got worried and phoned the police, who started to make investigations. The party, consisting of two tourists and their safari guide, had passed through Magadi on their way out, but no news of them had been heard since. They were in a well-equipped Land-Rover. If you go south towards Natron from Magadi it is straight forward down to Shombole and beyond for a certain distance, after which the track peters out. We had no idea where they had gone after this. Another pilot and myself took off at once at about 3.30 p.m. to make a preliminary aerial search at the request of the police. I knew this area quite well, not only from flying over it frequently, but also from a safari I had done with my family on the ground. Although within easy reach of Nairobi by air it is in fact very hostile terrain, hot, dry and often impassable.

We decided to fly down the track and then on down the east side of Lake Natron to see if there were any signs of the missing party. But first we landed at Magadi to get the latest news from the police. There was nothing new, so we sped on as there was not much time before dark to complete our search. The lake was still and appeared deserted of all human contact. It showed again its blood-red colour with circles of white soda which burns the skin if you try wading into the water. The flamingoes took off in their thousands and their shadows were reflected in the surface of the lake. Pelicans too showed off their flying ability, looking rather like the old Sunderlands of Coastal Command.

We arrived over the south end of Lake Natron and faced towards the mountain Ol Donyo Lengai, the volcano which stands as a sentinel guarding against any violation of this remote scene. All around were high mountains including Gelai, Kitembene, Loolmalasin and the crater of Ngoro Ngoro. The Maasai are the main tribe inhabiting this vast area and they move their cattle in and out according to the season, the rain and the grass. It is possible to get into this area from the south, though it is not easy and there are no tracks. There is tussock grass, sandy patches and deep ravines made by rain coming down off the mountains. These can be very treacherous and we had spent many hours digging our Land-Rover out of soft sand when we had explored the area from Mto wa Mbu. Really this is a place for two vehicles in convoy, because if you only have one and it gets stuck you are a long way from home and unlikely to be rescued. It is very hot, over 100°F., and there is no water until you get under the escarpment to the west. Here a fresh-water stream courses down through a rocky ravine and flows into the south-west corner of the lake.

I also remembered getting stuck on the shore of the lake which we had unwisely attempted to use as a road. The Land-Rover went through the soda crust and bellied down. It was a lengthy task to get it out as there were no stones to put under the wheels. We had jacked up our vehicle and laboriously put grass and matting underneath to get some purchase. We had been lucky to get out so I had no difficulty in envisaging a party getting permanently stuck in this unfriendly place. We decided to fly along the lake shore and then take a swing round Ol Donyo Lengai. There were no tracks on the lake shore, only a few zebra and thousands of water birds. We started to fly south and immediately realized how easy it would be to get lost and never be found. There was no sign around the mountain so we flew across to the river and then down it towards the lake. I was beginning to be very pessimistic about our mission as we banked again to scan another piece of country. Then I caught a glimpse of colour out of the corner of my eye. What could it be? I looked back and could see nothing again but the wasteland below. Yes, there it was again, a patch of orange. We flew over and saw that it was a tent laid out on the ground. Two figures were frantically waving. We had found them. Why were there two and not three people? I wrote and threw out a message which said, 'If you are all right put both hands in the air as we pass over.' Up went their hands as we circled back again. I then wrote out another message, 'Is the third person with you? If so, stick up your hands.' Again we got a positive response. We then decided to drop the food supplies we had brought. Out went the chocolate, the dried fruit and other provisions, quite enough to keep them going. Later we discovered that the safari guide had walked back to their Land-Rover which had become hopelessly stuck in soft sand in the bed of a dry river. It was eight miles from the place where we had seen them. They had been very wise and stayed close to the water which was their lifeline. A final message was dropped saying we would send in a land party as soon as it could be arranged. It was impossible to land anywhere near them so we could do no more.

With our mission successfully completed we left for home as dusk was falling. It was clearly important to reassure the relatives, inform the police and start organizing a land rescue party. This was all safely accomplished and we gained three grateful supporters.

In Africa, clouds, like the sun, are the constant companion of the pilot, part of his close environment, and he needs to study them to know what they hold in store for him. Eventually he develops a sixth sense about them based partly on knowledge, partly on experience and partly on intuition. I was flying once from Entebbe to Nairobi in an Aztec aircraft – the weather looked black and we knew from the weather reports that there were thunderstorms in all directions. In going into the cloud there was suddenly an awful clatter and the aircraft seemed to be being battered. I thought the windscreen was going to break as we realized that we were in a hailstorm. A quick 180° turn brought us out again into clear air; the windscreen was still intact but our nerves were badly jarred. I stored this up in my memory – hail in the tropics – look out.

Clouds can play funny tricks. They can hide hail, ice, hills, turbulence and a multitude of different conditions. They may not be solid but they can be very hostile. A countryside which is friendly, warm and hospitable on a clear day becomes a very different proposition with low cloud. All the hilltops disappear and landmarks vanish in the gloom; then every feature takes on a grey monochrome appearance and distinguishing marks fade into obscurity. Distance becomes deceptive; doubts begin to appear. Am I being blown off course? Surely that road should have been visible by now? The air is usually smooth, which helps and makes the flying more restful. Is that rain ahead? A grey curtain extends across my view but as I approach it is not as bad as I expected. I learn to probe the weather and often it looks better at close quarters than at a distance. Holes in the clouds open up and a way through can be found.

The man in charge of making an airstrip for us in Makiungu (a mission hospital near Singida in Tanzania) was convinced that clouds were solid and I felt it was my duty gently to disabuse him of this fact. When the great day arrived and the crowds gathered to see the Provincial Commissioner formally open the strip, I thought the best thing I could do was to take up those responsible for organizing the strip and give them a quick spin round in the aeroplane as a treat, and my friend, whose name was Augustus, was going to be my first passenger.

It was a happy day – the Irish nuns, who always exude an inner joy and serenity, were arranging a party afterwards at the hospital and there must have been a crowd of several thousand who had come to see the aeroplane, their friends and the Government officials. I was horrified to hear that I would be expected to say 'a few words' during the coming ceremony, so I frantically put together a few thoughts in very indifferent Swahili and went to greet the PC. We walked up the strip, which was a thousand yards long running east and west. The committee had carefully arranged to avoid the big white rocks which are such a feature of the country around Singida – the soil is sandy and often the crops are poor and a situation of semi-hunger exists much of the time. A piece of sisal string was attached between two poles at one end of the strip and this had to be cut by the PC as he finally opened the airstrip. First of all he made a speech congratulating all concerned for having given their labour in flattening the piece of land and working so hard. He gave them all a political pep-talk at the same time, which was expected of him. 'Kujenga Taifa' means in Swahili to build the nation, and what more suitable task than making an airstrip. We were told about 'self-reliance' and all the other slogans which could mean so much or so little depending on the context. At last his speech came to an end and it was my turn to stand on a chair and deliver my few halting words. I looked out over a sea of heads and felt for a moment what it must be like to be a demagogue and to sway crowds with passionate rhetoric. Despite my ineffectual and brief words of thanks to all who had helped with the strip, there was polite clapping all around as I stepped down to accompany the PC to the ceremony of cutting the tape. An amusing incident occurred at this moment; as the PC advanced, scissors in hand, to cut the tape and declare the strip formally open, we were dismayed to see that the sisal string had broken. Two stalwarts fortunately saw what had happened, quickly picked up the sisal string and knotted it together so that once again it formed a line across the end of the airstrip. The PC then duly cut it amid the laughter of the crowd. He, too, saw the funny side and from then onwards the evening was a great success.

It was my turn now to take up the committee members for a quick flight. Amid great excitement a large number of men pushed forward, all intent on getting into the plane. I fielded the first onslaught and explained I could take only three passengers at a time. I got Augustus to explain this and to organize the committee in groups of three.

Once this had been done, Augustus came forward and with two others we boarded the aircraft. Augustus sat by my side entranced with all the dials and knobs. I started up the engine and the noise helped to persuade the crowd to give me some room so that I could taxi down to the end of the strip and then take off over them and the hospital.

There were very few clouds that day so it meant climbing up to almost 9000 feet before I could line myself up to go through one. I saw Augustus grow pale under his dark skin. I tried to calm him, as I didn't want him opening the door and trying to get out at the critical moment. We entered the white fleecy cumulus cloud and shortly afterwards emerged in the bright blue sky again. Augustus was visibly shaken and started talking to his friends in the back seat in an animated fashion. When we landed, Augustus rushed off to his other friends and I could see him gesticulating wildly and pointing to the sky. How he explained that clouds were not after all solid, I shall never know.

This story about the clouds has always been in my mind, because although they are not solid, they manage to block all vision and as such they form a real barrier in the world of flying. Flying in clouds on instruments is done all the time every day, but in places where there are no navigational aids it is not advisable to come down through clouds blind and simply hope for the best. Without accurate information on the ground about cloud ceilings, it may

be very unwise to commit yourself to making a descent in moun-
tainous areas. In the months of July and August Nairobi is
notorious for low stratus cloud in the mornings and all local pilots
know the problems involved. I remember trying to get into Wilson
Airport early one morning from the farm. I got clearance to enter
the zone special VFR (visual flight rule) and was making my way
at about fifty feet above the ground. I thought I knew the area
fairly well but it is amazing how low cloud can confuse you.
I had tried once to turn and get out of the control zone again,
but the low cloud had come in behind me and I had had to make
another rapid turn to remain in sight of the ground. I called the
controller at Wilson Airport for what is called a QDM, which is
the course I had to steer to come out over the airfield. I was told
to steer 355°. I asked what the weather was like over the field
and he told me he could not see the runways. This was not very
encouraging. It was getting worse than when I had asked previously. I saw the game-park fence and knew I was now over
the field.

'Can I land on runway 32?' I said over the radio.

'Land on any runway you can see,' came back a cheery
Canadian voice. 'No one else is flying.'

He was trying to keep up my spirits and also point out kindly
that perhaps I was unwise to be flying at all. I had slowed right
down to 80 m.p.h. and had full flap down and my landing lights
on. The visibility cleared momentarily and I saw runway 32 on
my right. I must get in first time because I could not fly farther
without committing myself to cloud and the hangars were straight
ahead. I did a quick turn to the right and then to the left to line
up with the runway and put the aircraft down quickly. I had
three hundred yards left of the runway before going into the
fence and the main road. I saw the lights of cars crossing at right
angles to my path up the runway. The brakes were working well,
and as I turned off the runway I heaved an enormous sigh of relief.
I had frightened myself badly and before I switched off the engine
I vowed I would try not to get myself into such a position again.
I haven't succeeded but I have become more cautious and I hope
a little more cunning. I walked over to the tower to thank my
Canadian friend for his help in getting me in, and to apologize
for what was bad airmanship. I should have turned back before
and not put my head into such a noose. The Canadian smiled

ruefully and said, 'On a morning like this just remember the old adage – no see, no fly.'

I had once been told by an experienced pilot that flying consisted of frightening yourself stiff every three months with a period of relative calm in between. This is not a bad description and could be applied equally well to driving on the roads. On one occasion I was flying to Bukoba on the western shore of Lake Victoria. It was a grey day with a lot of rain about but it seemed to be well broken up and I unwisely didn't give it enough thought. I was on a journey to work at a mission hospital. I flew from Nairobi and dropped a parcel at Shirati on the east coast of the lake as this was scarcely out of my way to Bukoba. The flight across the lake was about one hundred and thirty-five nautical miles, which would take me just over the hour. The first half of the lake crossing was uneventful but clearly the weather was deteriorating and the rain became more and more solid. There was no way of ascertaining the latest weather at Bukoba although I had looked at the forecast before I started and there was no radio there and no beacon or other navigational help. I remembered an experienced pilot telling me that there was always a cumulo-nimbus cloud sitting out in the lake to the south of Bukoba in the mornings, so I planned to hit the west coast of the lake to the north and then fly down the coast to Bukoba.

I started to notice a few flashes of lightning but kept to my course, which was almost due west, and flew on. The height of the lake above sea level is 3750 feet and I had set my altimeter at Shirati which is at lake level. Now I began to have difficulty in distinguishing the grey of the cloud from the grey of the water and my forward view was almost entirely obliterated by the rain, but I could see a little through my side window. I have always preferred to fly in rain than low cloud but of course often you have both together. Once I did a 180° turn to see what it looked like behind me. It was no better, though I knew that if I flew sufficiently far to the east I would probably finally break out of the bad weather. I turned round again some fifty feet above the water and determined to fly on for a further ten minutes when I reckoned I should see the coast. I was well aware that there are times when it is best to swallow one's pride and retreat but on this occasion the easiest way out seemed to continue as I was getting close to my destination.

I realized that I was beginning to sweat and hold the controls tighter than I needed to. I tried to relax and yet be totally vigilant. The weather outside got darker and darker and the lightning became vicious at times. Only a few more minutes and I should see the coast. Perhaps 'see' was not quite the word. The hills rise quite steeply from the lake around Bukoba and I was anxious not to head straight into them in view of my total inability to see forward. I was already three minutes over my estimated time when I sensed I was nearing the shore; I turned through 90° towards the south and as I turned I thought I saw a denser shadow which could have been the hills. I could still see the surface of the lake dancing with the rain. I peered out by leaning across the co-pilot's seat to the right. Yes, there was the coast, indistinct but enough to satisfy me. I flew on south looking for Bukoba. I began to worry about the surface of the runway. I knew I would have to come in from the lake direction because I had no hope of approaching from the hills to the west as they rose quite sharply from the western end of the runway.

By now I was really frightened and my visibility was almost nil. I contemplated going back across the lake as I had enough fuel to do this. Perhaps the weather had closed in at Shirati and Mwanza and it might be equally bad that side. Indecision was beginning to sap my remaining courage. What a stupid way to die, I thought. Finally an icy calm took over and I steadied my mind, as I instinctively knew that if I panicked now I was a dead man. Then I caught a glance of the first buildings on my right. I decided to open the side window and turn the plane round so that I could watch the shore from my seat on the left side of the aircraft. I turned away from the shore to avoid the hills and did my 180° turn until I was flying north. The buildings had vanished so I edged my way closer in to where I thought the shore was. As I did so I saw the end of the runway which stopped at the lake. It appeared to be almost entirely under water but I was past the end of it before I had a chance of turning and landing.

I had determined now that I would land on the runway whatever its condition because the alternatives were worse, so I turned out into the lake again at once, since I knew I must stay as close to the airport as possible in case the low cloud cleared momentarily and gave me a better view. By now I was flying with my eyes standing out on stalks trying to pierce the darkness and rain.

I slowed down, put on full flap and approached the point where I thought the runway was, coming once again from the south. This time I knew I must get down as I was having great difficulty in fighting the panic which threatened to overwhelm me. My guardian angel had been working overtime and I was still alive. Yes, there was the shore again and a few buildings. I turned to the west and arrived on the runway about one-third down its length. Now was the moment; I had to get down because with the hills at the other end I had no chance of going round again. I closed the throttle, looked out of my small open window and resigned myself to whatever was in store for me. My wheels hit the ground and an enormous deluge of water was thrown up over the windscreen. I could see nothing but I stopped in a very short space. As the water cleared I saw that the aircraft was miraculously on the runway and appeared undamaged. I shut off the engine as I could not see where to taxi and the water was so deep. I began to realize that I was still alive and at that moment nothing else mattered but the feeling of relief.

I got out under the wing and looked back from where I had come out of the gloom. The water poured into my shoes but I scarcely noticed this. There was not a soul in sight. I took out the key, locked the door and started to walk in the direction of the airport offices which I could dimly see ahead of me. It was still pouring with rain and in a moment I was soaked. It was the most delicious drenching I have ever had. The realization that this particular ordeal was over was so great that I suddenly felt like singing. I clambered up the bank and out of a window of the offices stared three astonished black faces. What on earth was a drenched white man doing out there singing his head off? We always knew they were mad and this proves it, they seemed to say by their expressions. I was let in through the door and I imagine I must have looked an amazing sight as water ran off me on to the floor and I wiped my hair from my eyes and took a look round.

'Jambo,' I said.

No answer. Their jaws were still hanging open, until at last one African who seemed to me the man in charge said:

'*Wewe nane?*' 'Who are you?'

To tell the honest truth I didn't know who I was at that moment and the utter absurdity of the situation struck me so that all I could do was to laugh. It was probably rather a hysterical laugh but the ice was broken and soon we were fast friends and I was being peppered with questions. The only thing they refused to believe was that I had arrived by air; this was clearly impossible. The noise of the rain on the tin roof had drowned the noise of my engine as I had come in. It was still raining so hard that they couldn't see the aeroplane on the runway though I could distinguish it through the downpour. I was given a towel and I took off my shirt and rubbed myself down and then came the first cup of tea and with it my first feelings of remorse. I had put my head in a noose unnecessarily – another example of poor airmanship.

I had certainly scared myself stiff and remembering the statement about flying consisting of frightening oneself severely every three months followed by periods of relative calm, I was looking forward intensely to the latter.

I could not get any message through on the radio as there wasn't one. I decided to wait until the rain had abated, park the aircraft and then walk down to the town and try and establish contact. Later on I found my friends who had come to meet me. They found it difficult to believe, as I did myself, that I had come in through the storm. By lunch time the rain had stopped and I was able to go with my friends to the hospital and start the work I had come to do.

I soon recovered from the episode and I hoped that I had learnt something in this hard school which is the bush pilot's way of life. Since then I have, like most other pilots, had moments of acute fear and feelings of imminent disaster but they have been few and far between and quickly forgotten. I have had exactly the same feelings while ski jumping, mountain climbing and car rallying. I believe we get these sensations to enable us to react quickly. It is part of the very strong human instinct for survival. Calling this instinct into play is part of the response to those tingling moments of fear.

I must confess that no sixth sense warned me when I was operating in Nairobi one day and an urgent phone call came through from the farm. My next-door neighbour was on the phone.

'Mike, I've got some bad news for you,' he said. I waited for the next sentence with my heart in my mouth. What had happened? Was my family in some trouble?

'There has been a fire at your home and I'm afraid everything has been destroyed,' came the next announcement.

'Are the family all right?' I asked, scarcely daring to formulate the words.

'Yes. No one was in the house and the servants did what they could but it was impossibly hot. I am so sorry,' he said. 'I wanted you to know before you flew overhead and saw the smouldering ruin so you could at least be warned.'

'Thanks, John,' I said, 'it was very kind of you to have thought of it – I'm most grateful. I'll be down as soon as possible.'

I finished my operating list, but I couldn't help constantly thinking of what this would mean to Sue and the family. Where should we go for the night? Down to my daughter Janet's house, I imagined. As I left for Wilson Airport and clambered into my aircraft, I knew that the only thing that mattered was that everyone was alive and no one had been burnt. I thanked God for that.

I couldn't get the aircraft to go any faster and it seemed an age before Ol Molog came in sight. I could still see some smoke rising from the area where I knew our house was. Shortly afterwards I was overhead and looked down into what had been my home. There was nothing left except the fireplaces which survived because they were made of stone. The rest of the rambling old house had been made of wood with a cedar shingle roof. I saw a bath standing out in the open in an incongruous fashion.

I landed and was picked up by the family. Sue was, as always, calm and controlled, though I could see that the shock was still with her. I went up to the site and as we drove I heard the story. Sue had been out at lunch twenty miles away with Janet. There had been an explosion in the kitchen and the servants rushed over to see a fire getting out of control. They did all they could but there was a strong easterly wind blowing and everything was tinder dry. Bravely they rushed into the house and threw a few things out before the ammunition began going off, but they got the guns out first.

My imagination always leads me to the scene where our gallant servants were trying to get our double bed out through the window. To an African a bed is very valuable, but perhaps we should have been better pleased if some of the smaller things like pictures and Persian rugs had caught their attention. Neighbours had kindly rushed to the scene and also rung Sue at Janet's house. Robin came up the road in record time; there was nothing he could do. Even the plastic hosing which had been used for spraying water on the fire finally melted from the heat. We think that the gas stove was leaking and the gas crept across the floor until it was ignited by the flame of the paraffin refrigerator. After the explosion the fire took very quickly and became overwhelming in a short space of time.

I stood with Sue and gazed into the ruins. The silver had been melted into a shapeless mass by the heat of the fire. The pictures, the books, the gramophone records, our photograph albums, a book I was writing, all our clothes, linen, crockery, cutlery, Persian rugs and our precious sentimental things had all gone up in smoke. Years after the fire, indeed up to the present time, we keep on remembering things we had lost in this conflagration.

Life had to go on and sadly we turned away and made our way down to the small house on the farm which was occupied by Robin and Janet. They kindly moved out of their room and we all fitted in somehow to the small house. I started to grieve for my books and the few precious possessions I had. Sue was tremendously brave and we ended up laughing about our predicament – what else was there to do? We made a list of things to go and buy in Moshi the following day, toothbrushes, shoes, a saucepan or two, a jersey – just enough to keep us going while we took stock.

It had been a lovely home to us because we had built most of it ourselves and we had seen it grow with the family. Sue had designed a really comfortable living-room some thirty feet long and at one end had been an enormous plate-glass window with a bench window-seat from which you could absorb the panoramic view. I remembered the first tragedy surrounding this window. With great care we had ordered this vast piece of plate glass and months later it came up on a lorry. Sue hurried out to help unload it, only to find that the glass had been laid on its face and not stood up on its side. Of course it was in small pieces and a total loss. It took another few months before another piece could arrive.

I thought of my collection of mountaineering books, the St Matthew passion records; Mark, our eldest son's butterfly collection was another great sorrow; twenty-five boxes of beautiful butterflies were consumed in the fire, and all the other elements which had made our home. The house had an essential quality which reflected Sue's personality and taste and it was also a piece of art because she possessed to a high degree that sense of colour and design which lifts all she does above the humdrum and the commonplace.

When the immediate grief was over, in a strange way, we found the experience a salutary one. It was like having a giant spring-clean or having someone come in and send all your things to the jumble sale. We felt free to start again uncluttered by material possessions of any kind. Well, the first thing to do was to get those toothbrushes and start again.

Volumes could be written about the life at Ol Molog, but having recently had to leave it as a result of it being bought by the Tanzanian Government, I no longer have the wish to prolong the agony of separation. It was a wonderful time and we vowed never to have any regrets or bitterness. Ol Molog owed us nothing and we were only thankful for having been allowed to live there for twenty precious years.

I realize now – and it took a journey of twelve thousand miles round Canada and a total change of scene to make me appreciate it – that apart from problems of distance the impact of western culture is central to everything I have ever tried to do in Africa. In some ways it is a sobering thought and I have needed to thrash it out in my mind as it has been bothering me subconsciously for a long time.

A hundred years ago when the first missionaries and colonizers were moving into new lands, they had no doubt that what they were doing was right. This lack of doubt perhaps helped them to accomplish the amazing feats of exploration and undergo the hardships which were part of their everyday lives. This confidence in their cause remained a dominant factor until the First World War. Since that time there has been a gradual falling away of the confidence, and doubt and guilt have taken its place. What was it that gave rise to this change? It must have been a number of factors and perhaps we are still too close to the events to be able to take an objective view. Clearly our faith in the mission of western civilization was dealt a series of body blows in the war years. The building of western empires had, in fact, been in the hands of relatively few people and most of these were from the upper educated classes. India was ruled for two hundred and fifty years by a handful of men, about ten thousand in number at any one time. The Christian religion began to lose some of the fervour engendered in the days of Moody and Sankey, but perhaps most important of all was the reaction in the colonial people themselves. It seemed that they were happy to enjoy the technology which had been brought to them and there was a clamouring for education and better health, but it seems now the the cultural change was not very great and the colonizers began to feel that the colonized were ungrateful and that they were misunderstood. The feeling for independence grew, and more and more the western influence was rejected. It is difficult to discover a single example of where the new western civilization has been happily absorbed into the peoples of the developing world. It has always produced antagonism and has demoralized many people along the way. Some have been totally overwhelmed and turned into drunkards and spivs as their old way of life was destroyed and they had nothing to hang on to. Many of those who brought in western civilization were unimaginative, even if their intentions and motives were good.

In the north of Canada, which I visited recently, it seems as if the native peoples have suffered the same fate. Their old way of life has been interfered with and their roots pulled up. It is not surprising that they have taken to alcoholism. A cynic told me in Inuvik at the mouth of the Mackenzie River that the three great diseases of the north were alcoholism, venereal disease and welfare.

It is possible to kill someone with kindness. If an out-of-work Indian receives $400 welfare per month, it is not surprising that he drinks himself to death. No one with whom I spoke seemed to be able to produce a solution, though they all recognized and admitted the situation. It seems as though generosity can be misplaced if it destroys a man's will to work and uproots him from his traditions and disciplines. The welfare state in Britain could be said to show some of the same effects.

I was convinced that the health care I saw was being delivered in a generous and efficient way by kindly people who had excellent motives, and yet if we look at the overall result brought about by contact with our civilization, we must be very concerned at what we see.

So what do we do? Do we retire and leave them to their own devices? Can we modify successfully what is being done to produce a better answer?

I wish I knew, because it is of great significance in all humanitarian and development work around the globe. Most people shy away from discussing this issue and carry on blindly with what they are doing. It is certainly no place for moralizing.

I think the sickness in our civilization is very deep and we shall be unable to help other people until we cure our own ills. 'Physician, heal thyself.' I believe that Albert Schweitzer in his later years was tortured by the recognition that our civilization had taken several wrong turns. He used to say, 'I didn't come to change Africa, I came to serve Africa.' And this precept was basic to much of what he did. Many people may disagree with what he did but he realized that only example had any lasting effect. Perhaps it is because we do not do what we say that is at the root of our dilemma.

This is as close as I can get to a solution to this enigma. I do know, however, that the people who have made a lasting contribution in the developing world are the ordinary people who believe in what they are doing and live by ethical standards which are difficult to fault. The missionaries may have made many mistakes but they have lived out their faith and I have witnessed in many places the effect they have had. The African Christian is coming to the testing time when he has to stand up for his belief in the face of persecution and once again history will be seen to repeat itself. So I come to the conclusion that this generation has to make the choice as every other generation has had to in the past.

Epilogue: Pilgrim's Progress

As the communications grew so AMREF grew, supported by generous people both in and outside Africa. In a strange way people benefit from being part of an ideal which comes true. It restores faith in human enterprises. All along I was lucky with my friends and the contacts which I was fortunate enough to make. The team began to grow and flourish and whereas in the early days I had been director, office boy, pilot, doctor and fund-raiser, gradually people came along who did each of these jobs better than I could. To run a successful organization, you have to make yourself dispensable, and the quicker the better. So often the man who has the idea to start a venture is not the man to run it. I was acutely conscious of this, but so grateful to my friends for not reminding me of it too often. I suppose over the years I have made every major mistake it is possible to make, but I flatter myself that I learnt from these mistakes by admitting them.

I found, as everyone does who starts on such a venture as ours, that you will be criticized every inch of the way. There are the gloom spreaders – how are you going to pay for it? It has never been done before and it cannot be done in Africa – you do not understand the difficulties and so on *ad nauseam*. This used to worry me – now it bounces off my thick skin without leaving a mark.

I was much amused on one occasion to be sent the following

extract from a letter written by Voltaire on 4 October 1771 to Madame La Marquise du Deffand which puts the whole matter in a nutshell :

As soon as one wishes to do any good act, one is sure to make enemies. Should one render a service of any kind whatever, one can be certain of meeting with people who will try and crush you. Whether you write prose or verse, or you build a town, it is all the same; you will arouse a persecuting jealousy. There is only one way to escape from that harpy; never write anything but your epitaph, never construct anything except a monument for your tomb and get inside it as quickly as you can.

You just have to go slowly on doing what you believe you should be doing. It is hard at times. I was so encouraged to read the following quotation in a friend's office on the fifty-fifth floor of the Rockefeller building in New York. It must have helped many people who read it. It was written by Theodore Roosevelt :

It is not the critic who counts, not the man who points out how the strong man stumbled or where the doer of deeds could have done them better. The credit belongs to the man who is actually in the arena, whose face is marred by dust and sweat and blood, who strives valiantly, who errs and comes short again and again, who knows the great enthusiasm, the great devotions and spends himself in a worthy cause, who at the best knows in the end the triumph of high achievement, and who at the worst, if he fails, at least fails while daring greatly, so that his place shall never be with those cold and timid souls who know neither victory nor defeat.

Heroic stuff and it may be presumptuous to place oneself in the arena but this quotation made me think that perhaps persistence was a virtue to cultivate. Some people might call it obstinacy or bloody-mindedness, but it comes in useful at times. By all means take heed of the criticisms but carry on doing what your conscience tells you is right. In the end you win over some of your critics but of course some go on carping and perhaps it is good that they should, for it keeps you on your toes.

I have written about a few episodes with which I have been connected along the road, and as I come to the end I wonder whether it is possible to draw any conclusions. I do so with great humility but also with the knowledge that in a very uncertain world it is perhaps important to pin one's colours to some mast, but anything I can say as a comment on life as I see it must suffer from many inadequacies. I was brought up in the tradition that it is really not good form to discuss politics, money or religion and if you want to keep your friends this may still be good advice. But surely these topics are really the meat and essence of life, and if we refuse to discuss them because we are going to hurt somebody's feelings, then we should retire to a Trappist monastery.

Politics, in most places, have fallen into disrepute of late as the democratic tradition has been seen to falter in many places. We are hard on our politicians while on all sides you hear that politics is a dirty game. Has it always been so? Need it be? I do not know, but I sense that often the electorate is underestimated by the politicians. They could stand a little more truth and a little less bluff. There are instances where the constitution of a democratic state has been wonderfully upheld. The resignation of President Richard Nixon took place as a direct consequence of the press keeping on the trail and, finally, politicians standing up for the constitutional process. It was a fine day when this happened as it helped a great deal to restore faith in the legality of elected Government.

However, there are many examples where this has not occurred. Africa abounds with examples of where the country's legal constitution has been thrown out of the window when it suited the book of the clique in power. It was an article of faith in British colonial times that you only had to adopt the Westminster system and everyone would live happily ever after. This has not occurred and perhaps it was the height of naïveté to believe that it could have succeeded. The dictatorships and military Governments which took over in so much of Africa could hardly have come as a surprise to anyone who had lived there any length of time. And now, particularly in Britain and elsewhere, it is fashionable to denigrate the Government of South Africa. This is fair enough if you disagree with the philosophy of apartheid as most of us do. But it is the height of hypocrisy to remain silent about certain African countries which practise things which are just as bad, if not worse, than what goes on in South Africa. In fact, we allow a double standard, depending on who is involved, and it is this which sticks in so many people's throats. To his great credit, it was President Julius Nyerere who pointed this out and perhaps it was better said by an African, particularly one with such integrity. Black-white situations may be full of problems, but so also are black-black and white-white situations.

There were thirty-eight military coups in Africa during the first few years of African independence. Often the military take over when the occupation of the civil power has fallen into such disrepute that the population becomes totally disillusioned. At the start the military may be able to tidy things up and put down corruption, but usually they have little concept about the administration of a state and soon they find that people cannot live on slogans and manifestos, and repressive measures become tougher and tougher until there is another coup and the cycle starts again.

In the dictatorships of Africa, it is possible to see many of the mistakes which dictators in Europe made in the 1930s. One of the most insidious is the non-stop Government propaganda which so many states put out, and which the dictator and his clique finally begin to believe themselves. No one will tell them the real truth about what is going on in the country because they are afraid for their own necks, so eventually decisions are being made with little reference to the conditions which actually pertain. The dictator is surrounded by yes-men and sycophants, and then in the end he is signing his own death warrant because he is unaware of the opposition about which even his secret police will not tell. It is a common and disastrous pattern and it is played out only too often.

Fortunately, for a time, the colonialists and imperialists could be blamed for every error but this practice is wearing a little thin and the more outspoken African politicians admit that it is time they stood on their own feet and accepted some of the responsibility of failures themselves. Doubtless the colonial régimes were not without blame. Lack of imagination was perhaps their greatest failure. On the whole, integrity in public service, good administration and justice were the hallmarks of the British colonial era. Some of them were arrogant and treated the Africans as second-class citizens in their own countries. Sometimes their wives may have been a problem – 'the Memsahib mentality'. However, there is no doubt that the British sent to the colonies some of their finest and most dedicated men who gave of their best and it was a privilege to have known some of them. They were not exploiters, their salaries were often ridiculously low and they set an example of administration of which any country could be proud. It may be unpopular to voice these opinions at this time, but I believe it to be the truth.

Doubtless more could have been done and should have been done during the colonial period. With hindsight this becomes more apparent. No country is ever ready for independence and therefore it is vital to make the transference of power while good-will exists and to do so with a definite staged plan which both sides can understand. People only become responsible when they start to exercise responsibility. The retreat is always considered the most difficult military manœuvre and so it proved in the case of the Empire. Despite many setbacks in many places it has been successful. It is very clear that African countries prefer to rule themselves and it would be strange if they did not. I have heard Africans say in essence, 'We would rather rule ourselves badly than be ruled by you' – a very natural sentiment with which I can sympathize entirely.

It has been intensely interesting to have lived through the colonial period, the stages to independence and finally independence itself and the post-independence era. Everyone who has the interests of Africa at heart wishes to see the new young African Governments succeed as they are thrown into the mêlée of of modern politics and international relations. No one will expect miracles and many mistakes have and will be made. African Governments are not alone when it comes to error.

The Africans, although very different in different parts of Kenya, have certain great attributes which will stand them in good stead as they try to plot a course for their future. They are courteous, good humoured, trusting, fatalistic and have an ingrained sense of what is right. Civilizations have come and gone and perhaps it will be the African's turn in time to make a major contribution to human progress, but it is far too early to say.

Most African states profess to be socialist, but this generic term is used in so many different contexts that it has almost become meaningless. I feel that socialism has done a job over the past fifty years but that it is running out of steam. Equality of opportunity could be agreed to as a principle by many but it will never lead to equality of results. Once a system becomes based on envy or class hatred as certain socialist states are today, then production will suffer and the standard of living will go down for all.

As the modern international scene is so complex, there has to be a certain amount of central Government control. The *laisser-faire* method cannot any longer cope, but this is no excuse for too much Government with top-heavy bureaucracy. Nationalization is a highly controversial concept which has been shown to work under certain conditions and which has been an abysmal failure in others. Nationalized agriculture produces far less than the free-enterprise system of, say, the USA. In parts of Africa where Governments have interfered with agricultural practice, the scene is dismal in the extreme. Why should Government be a good farmer? Why should it do it better than the man who is brought up to it and has the real personal interest in making it succeed? He knows and cares for the land in a way that no Government can hope to do.

How are we to overcome the problem that nationalization tends to lead to more bureaucracy, more inefficiency, higher cost and appalling waste? It is possible to make out a case for the nationalization of public utilities, even if Government has to subsidize them. Perhaps the mixed economy where certain industries are run by Governments and others are left in private hands may prove to be the best solution during the coming years. If we take 'health' as an industry, it is difficult at this juncture to see how anyone is going to afford it. Already, even in the USA, certain aspects of health, such as mental health, are highly subsidized by the Federal Government. At the moment, the politicians are terrified to say no to the demands for medicine in all its forms, though it is clear that a point must be reached where a ceiling is put on these expenses. The cost is likely to increase rather than diminish. One way in which it could be met at the present time is to reduce the enormous defence budgets and arms industry of the major powers. A recent pamphlet put out by agencies dealing with the poverty of the developing world quotes the following horrifying statistic that the world spends on defence as much as the combined budgets for education and health. This draws in stark outline what the arms race is doing to destroy the chances of the developing world getting on its feet.

I left Canada with another view of what modern technology can bring us in the field of medicine. Using the satellite system it is possible for a consultant to sit at his desk in Montreal and discuss and advise on the treatment of a patient thousands of miles away. The patient, his X-rays, his ECG (electrocardiogram) can be shown on the television screen in his consulting-room and he can discuss the history and the signs and symptoms with whoever is attending his patient on the spot. He can thus make his skilled knowledge available to those who need it far away in the remote parts of the country. At the present time this must be an expensive service beyond the bounds of possibility for the developing world, but it is possible to see a glimpse of what the future may hold for us.

This and other journeys to the remote parts of the world helped to give me some perspective of the overall problem which would have to be tackled if health care was one day to be brought to the places where it was so urgently needed. They helped, too, to convince me about the type of services which were most required. It was clear that a great deal could be done at the grass-roots level by the application of a little common sense, and that expensive hospitals and specialists were an unnecessary luxury and even a burden in many places. The example of the 'barefoot' doctor in China has shown what can be done, thought it is far from perfect. As I thought about these matters the key seemed to lie in the training of a cadre of people who could live happily in the peripheral areas of the world and concentrate on the basic health problems. This is easier said than done, because the tendency is the other way round, with people wanting to crowd into the urban areas. It has now been shown in many places in the world that the training itself has to be done at the periphery and not at the centre, and that the people best fitted for this task have to be from the local population itself. Supervision of these people has to be a priority so that standards and discipline are maintained, while refresher courses help to keep up interest and morale.

It is not going to be easy for anyone to spread the concept of primary health care but a new enthusiasm is being born for it, and the emphasis from a growing number of authorities is moving in its favour. Communities are going to have to do more to save their health by their own efforts.

Although we were told by Marx that in the communist state after an initial period 'the state would wither away', we have in fact seen the very opposite – the state has become all-powerful and repressive, so that little or no individual freedom is left.

I believe in individual responsibility wherever possible. Too much is shirked and the buck is passed to 'them', which means the authorities. The welfare state has led to an erosion of initiative and incentive and this is very clear in the health field. In the final analysis, the crucial point in ideology is whether the state exists for the people or the people exist for the state; and it is to individual people we, as doctors, must always come back.

I was reminded of this a few days later back in Nairobi as I was driving down to the local shop to pick up a few household things. I was going slowly and enjoying the freedom and peace of the holiday when I felt the car beginning to pull to the right and steer awkwardly. I stopped and got out and saw immediately that I had a puncture. I went to the boot to get out the jack and spare tyre when an African came up to me and said with a big smile, '*Jambo, Bwana* Michael.' I answered his greeting while looking at him closely.

'*Unakumbuka mimi, Bwana?*' he said, which means, 'You remember me?' Well, I did remember him but I could not remember his name or when I had met him. He saw that I was puzzled and went on to tell me that he had been a patient of mine in a hospital in Nairobi in 1952. I was still puzzled, then he turned round and pulling his coat collar down he showed me a big scar on the back of his neck. Slowly it began to dawn that this was my old patient Samuel Kamau and the story came back to me.

He had been knocked down in a motor-car accident and had come in with a fracture dislocation of his neck and paralysis below his sixth cervical vertebra. I remembered his wide generous smile and the first time I had seen it when he was lying helpless in bed on that first evening. I had got him X-rayed and went down to see the films which showed the dislocation of his fifth cervical vertebra on his sixth. I took him to the theatre and made two small holes through the outer table of his skull above his ears and put in a device called a 'Clutchfield clamp'. On returning him to the ward, we tipped his bed with his head up and feet down and attached some weights to the clamp. This had the effect of stretching the neck by means of the weights pulling one way and the weight of his body the other. It sounds like a crude piece of medieval torture but in fact is not as agonizing as it sounds. I had left him that evening under sedation and over the next few days new X-rays showed the position of his neck improving, but more startling than that he began slowly recovering from his paralysis and loss of sensation. We had got him under treatment in time. His spinal cord had been contused but not irreparably damaged. He was always a delight to visit as he was invariably cheerful and instead of me having to cheer him up, he cheered me up.

We found eventually that he had an unstable neck and that when the traction was reduced his troubles recurred. This necessitated a bone graft of his neck. The day came for the operation, blood had been cross-matched for him, and with his clamp still in place we turned him over on the operating table, after putting him to sleep, and opened his neck in the region of the fracture dislocation and dissected the muscles away both above and below the injury.

Having made a bed for the bone grafts a tourniquet was applied to his leg and long pieces of bone removed from one shin bone and placed in his neck. The wound in his leg was closed and dressed and the tourniquet removed. Little chips of bone which had also been taken from the leg were fitted into the jigsaw puzzle in his neck. The muscles were closed over the graft and the neck wound sutured. With great care we turned Samuel over on his back, returned him to the ward and fixed him once again to his traction apparatus.

As the weeks went by and Samuel began to mend, we were able eventually to dispense with the clamp. He was a marvellous patient. He co-operated with the physiotherapists and moved his arms and legs as the strength returned. He needed no encouragement as he was the sort of man who wanted to get out and about again and nothing was going to stop him. If anything, I had to admonish him for doing too much too quickly. Then the day came to prop him up and instead of looking at the ceiling he was able to look around the ward: the smile grew broader and his eyes lit up with excitement. And so Samuel eventually got out of bed and started walking. At first he needed help and support from crutches but soon he was using sticks and finally nothing at all. I had seen him a few times in out-patients afterwards, but finally I lost contact with him.

Here, twenty-three years later, was my old friend helping to change my wheel. The task was accomplished and I ran Samuel to his destination. He shook my hand till I thought it would come off. I turned my car round to head towards home and out of the corner of my eye I saw Samuel giving me a final salute.